TREATING TRAUMATIZED CHILDREN

TREATING TRAUMATIZED CHILDREN

A Casebook of Evidence-Based Therapies

Edited by

Brian Allen
Mindy Kronenberg

THE GUILFORD PRESS
New York   London

© 2014 The Guilford Press
A Division of Guilford Publications, Inc.
72 Spring Street, New York, NY 10012
www.guilford.com

Printed in the United States of America

This book is printed on acid-free paper.

Last digit is print number: 9 8 7 6 5 4 3 2 1

The authors have checked with sources believed to be reliable in their efforts to provide
information that is complete and generally in accord with the standards of practice that
are accepted at the time of publication. However, in view of the possibility of human error
or changes in behavioral, mental health, or medical sciences, neither the authors, nor the
editors and publisher, nor any other party who has been involved in the preparation or
publication of this work warrants that the information contained herein is in every respect
accurate or complete, and they are not responsible for any errors or omissions or the
results obtained from the use of such information. Readers are encouraged to confirm the
information contained in this book with other sources.

Library of Congress Cataloging-in-Publication Data

Treating traumatized children (Allen)
  Treating traumatized children : a casebook of evidence-based therapies / edited by Brian
Allen and Mindy Kronenberg.
    p. ; cm.
  Includes bibliographical references and index.
  ISBN 978-1-4625-1694-0 (hardback : alk. paper)
  I. Allen, Brian, 1979– editor.   II. Kronenberg, Mindy, 1975– editor.   III. Title.
  [DNLM: 1. Cognitive Therapy—methods.   2. Parent–Child Relations.   3. Stress
Disorders, Post-Traumatic—therapy.   4. Child.   5. Evidence-Based Practice.   6. Infant.
WM 172.5]
  RJ505.C63
  618.92′891425—dc23
                                                                                    2014016174

*In memory of Patricia Van Horn, a beloved teacher
whose wisdom and dedication are cherished*

*Her work on behalf of children and families
will inspire generations of therapists to come.*

About the Editors

Brian Allen, PsyD, is a clinical psychologist, Director of Mental Health Services at the Center for the Protection of Children at the Penn State Hershey Children's Hospital, and Assistant Professor of Pediatrics and Psychiatry at the Penn State Hershey College of Medicine. Dr. Allen's research interests include the dissemination and implementation of evidence-based treatments for children who have experienced maltreatment and trauma, understanding the developmental impact of childhood trauma, and the assessment and treatment of children with sexual behavior problems. He has written numerous articles for peer-reviewed scientific journals and is a frequent presenter at conferences related to trauma and child maltreatment. Dr. Allen regularly consults with clinicians on the implementation of trauma-focused cognitive-behavioral therapy and parent–child interaction therapy.

Mindy Kronenberg, PhD, is a clinical psychologist in private practice in Memphis, Tennessee. She is Adjunct Clinical Professor at Louisiana State University Health Sciences Center and an affiliate member of the National Child Traumatic Stress Network. Dr. Kronenberg's clinical and research interests include infant mental health, the assessment and treatment of trauma across the lifespan, psychological first aid, and the impact of trauma on young children. The author of numerous articles for peer-reviewed journals and book chapters, she frequently consults with agencies and clinicians regarding infant mental health, presents at conferences related to trauma and disaster, and is a national trainer for child–parent psychotherapy.

Contributors

Brian Allen, PsyD, Center for the Protection of Children, Penn State Hershey Children's Hospital, and Departments of Pediatrics and Psychiatry, Penn State Hershey College of Medicine, Hershey, Pennsylvania

Leslie Whitten Baughman, MA, Connect Counseling, Sacramento, California

Dawn M. Blacker, PhD, CAARE Diagnostic and Treatment Center, University of California, Davis, Children's Hospital, Sacramento, California

Joaquin Borrego, Jr., PhD, Department of Psychology, Texas Tech University, Lubbock, Texas

Alexandra Gibson, BA, Department of Psychology, Texas Tech University, Lubbock, Texas

Natalie Armstrong Hoskowitz, MA, Department of Psychology, Sam Houston State University, Huntsville, Texas

Chelsea Klinkebiel, MA, Department of Psychology, Texas Tech University, Lubbock, Texas

Mindy Kronenberg, PhD, independent practice, Memphis, Tennessee; Louisiana State University Health Sciences Center, New Orleans, Louisiana

Alicia F. Lieberman, PhD, Child Trauma Research Program, San Francisco General Hospital, San Francisco, California

Clare Lucas, MS, Children's Safe Harbor, Conroe, Texas

Michele M. Many, MSW, Department of Psychiatry, Louisiana State University Health Sciences Center, New Orleans, Louisiana

Benjamin E. Saunders, PhD, National Crime Victims Research and Treatment Center, Department of Psychiatry and Behavioral Sciences, Medical University of South Carolina, Charleston, South Carolina

Amy R. Sommer, MSW, Center for Early Relationship Support, Jewish Family and Children's Service, Waltham, Massachusetts

Eda Spielman, PsyD, Center for Early Relationship Support, Jewish Family and Children's Service, Waltham, Massachusetts

Alexandra Tellez, MA, Department of Psychology, Sam Houston State University, Huntsville, Texas

Anthony J. Urquiza, PhD, CAARE Diagnostic and Treatment Center, University of California, Davis, Children's Hospital, Sacramento, California

Patricia Van Horn, PhD, (deceased), Child Trauma Research Program, San Francisco General Hospital, San Francisco, California

Jeffrey N. Wherry, PhD, ABPP, DCAC Research Institute, Dallas Children's Advocacy Center, Dallas, Texas

Acknowledgments

This book was made possible through the support and encouragement of numerous individuals. We express our sincere thanks and appreciation to the skilled and knowledgeable clinicians and researchers who graciously gave their time and talents to contributing chapters and commentaries. We also wish to acknowledge the contributions of our colleagues and mentors within our immediate settings and across the United States who have assisted us in our professional development, practice, and scholarly pursuits. The dedication of these professionals to the validation, dissemination, and implementation of effective treatments for children who experience trauma and maltreatment is not only commendable, but also has a very real and profound impact on the lives of countless children and families.

Brian Allen would like specifically to thank Anthony J. Urquiza and Anthony Mannarino for taking a chance on an ambitious but naïve graduate student, and for their continuing support. Mindy Kronenberg would like to thank Joy Osofsky for introducing her to the field of infant mental health, fostering her growth as a clinician, and providing ongoing support and encouragement. She thanks Alicia F. Lieberman and the late Patricia Van Horn for trusting her to write about child–parent psychotherapy (CPP) and for creating a community that nurtures the growth of CPP clinicians. She would also like to thank her colleagues and friends Richard Costa, Amy Dickson, Joaniko Kohchi, Michele M. Many, Carmen Norona, Stacey Leakey, and Tamara Reed, who helped with editing and supported her efforts.

We would like to thank all of the children who participated in the case studies contained within this book. Although their identities are disguised, their participation in treatment and sharing of their stories not only improved the clinical skills of the clinicians with whom they worked, but also created a legacy of helping other children who came after them. Similarly, credit and recognition must be given to the supportive and dedicated families and caregivers of these children. Their involvement with and commitment to the children are irreplaceable, and there is no doubt that these children's lives are improved because of their efforts.

Last, it is only fitting that we thank those family members closest to us who provided our support network as we labored in the development of this book. Brian Allen wishes to thank his incredibly supportive and loving wife, Kristen; his amazingly spirited and wonderful daughter, Ashlyn; his two four-legged children, Barkley and Joey; his parents, Bill and Deborah Allen; and the rest of his family. Mindy Kronenberg thanks her mom and dad, Suzie and Joel Kronenberg, and her sisters, Becky Kronenberg and Erica McElroy, who have always provided unconditional love, support, and tolerance in all of her endeavors.

Preface

Mental health clinicians are under increasing pressure from health insurance companies, government agencies, and the general public to utilize evidence-based treatments (EBTs). EBTs, broadly defined, are psychotherapeutic techniques and protocols that have been submitted for empirical evaluation and demonstrated to be effective in reducing behavioral and/or emotional problems (Kazdin, 2008). Research indicates improved treatment outcomes when clinicians use EBTs compared to standard practice (Cary & McMillen, 2012; Weisz, Jensen-Doss, & Hawley, 2006).

The fields of child trauma and maltreatment have made great strides in developing and promoting EBTs. For instance, the establishment of the National Child Traumatic Stress Network (NCTSN) by the United States Congress in 2001 significantly increased the visibility and dissemination of EBTs for trauma-exposed children. A number of EBTs were identified, and significant resources were allocated to clinics and training centers across the country to promote their use. Moreover, the National Children's Alliance, the national accrediting agency for children's advocacy centers (CACs), recently revised their standards for the implementation of mental health services for maltreated children. The updated standards require that psychotherapeutic services be evidence based and informed by the latest research on childhood trauma and abuse.

Despite the empirical research on EBTs and the significant pressure exerted by policymakers to increase their use, it appears that changing the practices and attitudes of clinicians who serve trauma-exposed children is a slow process. A recent study found that out of 250 clinicians who provide services for maltreated children, less than one-third could identify more than one EBT (Allen, Gharagozloo, & Johnson, 2012). In addition, the majority of clinicians reported that they had received training in and regularly employed interventions that are not considered evidence based. Of those clinicians who did report using an EBT (specifically, trauma-focused cognitive-behavioral therapy), 33% self-reported a lack of fidelity to the treatment model (Allen & Johnson, 2012).

The lack of knowledge about and implementation of available EBTs may be due partially to dissemination methods that are not effective in reaching many mental health professionals. Allen and Armstrong (2014) found that clinicians identified case studies demonstrating the use of a treatment as the most desired form of evidence when selecting an intervention. Clinicians reported reading twice as many case studies as data-based research reports and generally obtained these case studies from published books. Although the developers of EBTs have successfully conducted several randomized clinical trials that demonstrate the superiority of EBTs over other treatments, they rarely provide complete case studies that discuss how these approaches are used. Rather, journal articles and published treatment manuals typically include only brief vignettes demonstrating the use of a particular skill or technique. Such examples, while clinically useful, are unable to fully explain how EBTs are used with culturally diverse, complex, or challenging families. Furthermore, the vignettes do not typically show modifications of the treatment protocol for specific clinical concerns or how to maintain fidelity to the model when modifications are made.

Our book attempts to address these concerns by providing complete case studies of EBTs as well as sufficient background for clinicians to understand an evidence-based approach to treatment. The book is divided into four parts. Part I provides an introduction to evidence-based treatments and has a chapter on the nature and development of EBTs and a chapter that highlights the critical role of assessment in providing evidence-based care. Parts II through IV cover three prominent EBTs for trauma-exposed children: trauma-focused cognitive-behavioral therapy (TF-CBT), child–parent psychotherapy (CPP), and parent–child interaction therapy (PCIT). Each part begins with an overview of the techniques and research base of the EBT and is followed by two chapters with case studies. In each case study, "real-world" clients are followed from intake to discharge, and the reader is able to examine how the clinician maintained fidelity to the treatment model and overcame typical barriers to treatment implementation, including cultural issues, unexpected clinical events, reluctant caregivers, and comorbid clinical presentations.

When constructing this book, we sought to dispel the following common myths about the implementation of EBTs in community settings:

- ***EBTs do not work in the "real world."*** Some clinicians believe that interventions developed by researchers in academic centers are not applicable in the "real world," where clients display multiple concerns and clinicians have limited time and resources. Each of the case studies explored in this book was written by a practicing clinician who treated the client in a community setting (e.g., community mental health center, drug treatment program, or children's advocacy center). In considering what kinds of cases should be included, we asked the clinicians to select cases that demonstrated clinical challenges and tested their skills. We did not want "textbook" cases.

• *EBTs are too rigid, or they employ a "cookbook" approach.* This is a common criticism of EBTs, but we hope that the diversity of case studies we present will demonstrate the flexibility of EBTs. We selected cases that highlight the clinicians' responses to unforeseen clinical events (e.g., a child placed in foster care during the course of treatment, or discord between caregivers). The cases also display the versatility of EBTs and their generalizability to a multitude of presenting histories, including sexual abuse, physical abuse, neglect, exposure to domestic violence, parental substance use, and involvement in the child welfare system. Among the presenting concerns of children in the case studies are posttraumatic stress, anxiety, depression, oppositional behavior, conduct problems, and aggression. The reader will quickly realize that no two cases are ever treated identically, even if the same EBT is employed.

• *EBTs are not useful for . . . (a specific demographic variable).* The three interventions discussed in this book were specifically chosen because they can be used with children from birth to 18 years. Furthermore, they are culturally sensitive, they demonstrate effectiveness in clinical trials with various ethnic groups, and they are employed with children and families from diverse ethnic, spiritual, and socioeconomic backgrounds.

• *EBTs are biased toward a specific theoretical approach.* Clinicians are often taught to develop a theoretical orientation or identity. If EBTs do not fit that approach, clinicians may hesitate to use them. However, EBTs originating from diverse theoretical perspectives are available. Collectively, the three interventions in this book originate from cognitive theory, social learning and behavioral theories, attachment theory, and psychodynamic theories.

• *Researchers do not listen to clinicians.* The clinician–researcher dialogue is an important, but often underappreciated, exchange that can improve our clinical techniques. Therefore, for each of the three EBTs, we identified researchers, who either developed or are professionally invested in the development and dissemination of the interventions. These experts provide commentaries at the end of each case study chapter and discuss how the particular case exhibits the application of the intervention with "real-world" clients. There is no "perfect case" nor perfect application of any given treatment approach; there is always more to learn, and the cases presented here are no exception. These expert commentators provide useful analysis regarding the delivery of the intervention and offer suggestions on how to enhance treatment. By virtue of the constructive feedback and numerous questions they receive from clinicians in the field, they have become disseminators of the collective clinical wisdom. We hope that readers will gain useful insights from the clinicians whose considerable talents are on display and from the commentators who discuss the case studies within the context of the larger knowledge base regarding the intervention.

Our goal in developing our book was to provide a solid foundation for both the novice clinician in the child trauma or maltreatment field and for the seasoned clinician who wants to learn more about EBTs and their applications. We encourage readers to view this book as an introduction to various EBTs and their use with trauma-exposed children and families, and not as didactic training in the use of the interventions. Each overview chapter includes resources that direct the reader to additional information about the EBTs discussed. The reader is encouraged to consult these resources to learn more about training programs and requirements for intervention implementation.

BRIAN ALLEN
MINDY KRONENBERG

REFERENCES

Allen, B., & Armstrong, N. E. (2014). Burden of proof: The evidence clinicians require before implementing an intervention. *Child and Adolescent Mental Health, 19*, 52–56.

Allen, B., Gharagozloo, L., & Johnson, J. C. (2012). Clinician knowledge and utilization of empirically supported treatment for maltreated children. *Child Maltreatment, 17*, 11–21.

Allen, B., & Johnson, J. C. (2012). Utilization and implementation of trauma-focused cognitive-behavioral therapy for the treatment of maltreated children. *Child Maltreatment, 17*, 80–85.

Cary, C. E., & McMillen, J. C. (2012). The data behind the dissemination: A systematic review of trauma-focused cognitive-behavioral therapy for use with children and youth. *Children and Youth Services Review, 34*, 748–757.

Kazdin, A. E. (2008). Evidence-based treatment and practice: New opportunities to bridge clinical research and practice, enhance the knowledge base, and improve patient care. *American Psychologist, 63,* 146–159.

Weisz, J. R., Jensen-Doss, A., & Hawley, K. M. (2006). Evidence-based youth psychotherapies versus usual clinical care: A meta-analysis of direct comparisons. *American Psychologist, 61,* 671–689.

Contents

PART I

FOUNDATIONS OF EVIDENCE-BASED TREATMENT

1

Understanding Evidence-Based Treatment for Trauma-Exposed Children

Definition, Development, and Misconceptions

Brian Allen

Few topics in the mental health field have generated more controversy in recent years than the progressively greater role of research in the development and implementation of treatment approaches. Numerous governmental agencies, insurance companies, and other third-party payers and policymakers are encouraging, and in some instances requiring, the use of research-supported interventions; however, critics have voiced numerous objections against the move toward a more empirically based approach to treatment. Complicating the issue are numerous misconceptions and confusion about the development of these interventions and how they are implemented in practice.

Perhaps the greatest confusion derives from the multitude of names and definitions that describe the movement toward the greater use of research in practice. Terms such as *evidence-based practice* and *evidence-based treatment* are often used interchangeably with little recognition that each term actually denotes a different idea of clinical practice. The research community itself is unable to agree on a single term and definition (Self-Brown, Whitaker, Berliner, & Kolko, 2012). This lack of terminological and definitional consensus has resulted in disagreements about which treatment techniques or packaged protocols possess adequate empirical support and are, therefore, appropriate for widespread implementation. Correspondingly, clinicians are often unsure about the interventions for which they should seek training (Allen, Gharagozloo, & Johnson, 2012) and may be confused and resistant when funders or agencies require that they change their practice to use specific evidence-based interventions.

DEFINING EVIDENCE-BASED TREATMENT

The most widely used term, *evidence-based practice* (EBP), typically represents "the integration of the best available research with clinical expertise in the context of patient characteristics, culture, and preferences" (American Psychological Association, 2006, p. 273). This definition recognizes the unique contributions of research-derived knowledge and clinical experience and emphasizes that treatment must be tailored for unique client considerations. By this definition, EBP is not a set of techniques or a manualized intervention, but rather encompasses a larger context that incorporates both clinician and client factors. EBP provides considerable clinician freedom to determine how these separate but related factors (research, clinical expertise, client characteristics) can be integrated to achieve the desired clinical outcome.

However, this general definition of EBP has not gone unchallenged. For instance, Baker, McFall, and Shoham (2008) noted that the American Psychological Association definition "equates the personal experiences of the clinician and client preferences with scientific evidence—a striking embrace of a prescientific perspective" (p. 84). The American Psychological Association definition may be exceedingly broad in defining EBP, placing each of the three components on equal footing. Technically, a clinician may use his or her expertise and judgment to decide what constitutes "best available research," continue practicing according to his or her own clinical preferences, and be in compliance with an EBP perspective. Given the broad nature of the American Psychological Association definition, it becomes very difficult, if not impossible, to specify what does and does not constitute EBP.

In contrast, an *evidence-based treatment* (EBT; also known as an *empirically supported treatment* or *empirically validated treatment*) is a specific intervention or sequence of techniques with documented ability to create therapeutic change in controlled clinical trials (Kazdin, 2008). The specification of a treatment manual provides the clinician with a structured treatment approach specifically designed for the presenting concerns of the client. The validation of the treatment model in controlled trials provides assurance that the intervention being employed is effective for treating the identified symptoms or problems.

Multiple agencies and organizations have completed intensive reviews of the scientific evidence to identify EBTs for specific emotional and behavioral problems. These reviews may employ different criteria, but generally agree that designation as an EBT requires (1) the treatment possesses a sound theoretical basis, (2) the treatment is clearly specified in a manual or book that describes how to implement each component, and (3) at least two randomized clinical trials demonstrate either the superiority of the treatment over an appropriate control group or results equal to those obtained by another EBT (California Evidence-Based Clearinghouse for Child Welfare, n.d.; Saunders, Berliner, & Hanson, 2004; Silverman & Hinshaw, 2008). The ultimate goal of identifying EBTs is to improve the dissemination and implementation of effective interventions, thereby improving the quality of service delivery (Addis & Cardemil, 2006; Gibbs & Gambrill, 2002). The process of evaluating and validating an intervention is explained in greater detail later in this chapter.

FACTORS AFFECTING TREATMENT OUTCOME

To understand the importance of EBTs, it is necessary to consider the many factors that affect successful treatment outcome. Asay and Lambert (1999) provide a useful framework by classifying these factors into four distinct categories: (1) client variables and extratherapeutic events, (2) expectancy and placebo effects, (3) therapeutic relationship, and (4) treatment techniques. Each of these factors is discussed next with respect to treatment outcomes for trauma-exposed children.

Client Variables and Extratherapeutic Events

It is generally believed that a significant portion of treatment outcome is *not* related to the events that occur during treatment sessions. Rather, unique strengths and experiences of the client, as well as events that occur outside of treatment, exert a profound influence on one's mental health. *Client variables* include individual, familial, cultural, or systemic factors specific to a given individual that influence the development, prevention, or amelioration of mental illness. For instance, a common finding is that children with supportive caregivers involved in treatment exhibit greater benefit from mental health interventions than children whose caregivers are not involved (Deblinger, Lippmann, & Steer, 1996; Dowell & Ogles, 2010). Another example is the repeated observation that children displaying more adaptive and effective coping skills following sexual abuse are less likely to develop significant emotional and behavioral problems (Shapiro, Kaplow, Amaya-Jackson,

& Dodge, 2012; Simon, Feiring, & Kobielski McElroy, 2010). Client variables also include the characteristics of one's trauma experience. In considering sexual abuse, more severe and chronic abuse tends to result in more significant psychopathology, as does a closer relationship between the victim and perpetrator (Yancey & Hansen, 2010). These few examples are illustrative; however, countless other client variables also are influential in determining treatment outcome.

Extratherapeutic events, defined as events that occur outside of treatment sessions, can exert a significant impact on mental health. Extratherapeutic factors include the passage of time, changes in school setting, changes in family structure (e.g., parental marriage or divorce), and other such events that affect the child's mental health. For instance, abused children are at significantly increased risk for experiencing future episodes of maltreatment, bullying in school, and other stressful or traumatic situations (Mohaptra et al., 2010; Villodas et al., 2012). These events may limit the rate of progress in treatment or exacerbate the concerns with which a child presents. Reducing or eliminating various extratherapeutic stressors (e.g., parental unemployment, medical illness) may improve a child's mental health irrespective of the treatment services provided.

These few examples are meant to demonstrate that a child's mental health, including response to trauma, depends on various factors; psychotherapeutic intervention is only one of a multitude of influences. Asay and Lambert (1999) suggest that many clinicians, particularly novice clinicians, may fail to recognize the significant impact that client variables and extratherapeutic events have on treatment progress, instead crediting their clinical skill or techniques for treatment success. Alternatively, clinicians may attribute treatment failure to these variables (e.g., client resistance, complexity of the case), preventing them from considering that their clinical skills or techniques were ineffective. Clinicians are encouraged to recognize the significant impact of client characteristics and extratherapeutic events at all stages of the treatment process, including treatment planning and posttreatment evaluation.

Expectancy and Placebo Effects

Many clinicians are familiar with the concept of the placebo effect, which occurs when an inert substance or procedure is delivered to the client who, by the very fact that he or she believes that the inert treatment will work, begins to show improvement. The placebo effect demonstrates the impact that one's perceptions or beliefs can have on emotional and physical well-being. The placebo is commonly used in clinical trials of psychotropic medications. In these trials, a group of patients receives the active drug (e.g., an antidepressant), and a second group of patients unknowingly receives an inactive substance (e.g., a sugar pill). This simple design allows researchers to determine whether the active drug creates improvement in the targeted outcome or whether the improved outcome is only associated with the belief that improvement should occur.

In psychotherapy, expectancy effects manifest in similar ways. Caregivers may bring a child to a mental health clinician because they believe that a trained professional is needed to assist with the child's difficulties. This creates an expectation, from the initiation of services, that treatment progress is possible and that the clinician treating the child is competent and able to help. Treatment progress with children is often evaluated by the feedback of caregivers, and expectancy effects may implicitly influence caregivers' report of symptoms. In addition, positive expectations of treatment appear to predict better treatment outcomes, more consistent participation and attendance at sessions, and greater compliance with homework assignments (Lewin, Peris, Bergman, McCracken, & Piacentini, 2011; Nock & Kazdin, 2001).

The use of a true placebo condition in psychotherapy outcome studies is rare. To approximate the process and conditions encountered by those receiving the target intervention under examination, the control group is more likely to receive a psychotherapeutic treatment believed to create minimal change (i.e., nondirective supportive counseling) or standard clinical services. These control conditions typically include providing a therapeutic rapport with a supportive clinician, resulting in the control group receiving the effects associated with the expectation of positive outcomes (i.e., the placebo or expectancy effect) as well as any additional benefit provided by the therapeutic relationship.

The Therapeutic Relationship

An effective therapeutic rapport has been long considered a foundational principle of psychotherapy. Clinicians learn early in training to establish a therapeutic relationship by responding to the client in an empathic and genuine manner while demonstrating unconditional positive regard, factors that Carl Rogers (1957) deemed necessary and sufficient for therapeutic change to occur. The therapeutic rapport, if effectively established, provides the client with a sense of trust and respect that allows him or her to feel valued and accepted.

Some approaches to child psychotherapy maintain that the therapeutic rapport is the primary facilitator of change in treatment. Proponents of these types of treatment, therefore, suggest that establishing and maintaining rapport should be the primary treatment technique utilized by the clinician. For instance, in child-centered play therapy (Axline, 1969) the clinician is instructed to provide a safe and supportive environment, allow the child to direct the activities of sessions, and provide empathic comments in response to the child's play. The theory is that providing a warm and supportive atmosphere will create a sense of safety for the child and thereby allow him or her to express and process troubling thoughts and emotions, either verbally or nonverbally through play. This processing of emotional material is thought to ameliorate the presenting concerns. Indeed, treatment outcome research suggests improvement of child emotional and behavioral concerns following the delivery of rapport-focused interventions (Bratton, Ray, Rhine, & Jones, 2005).

Remembering the impact exerted by client variables, extratherapeutic events, and expectancy and placebo effects on treatment outcome, the impact of therapeutic rapport must be examined in context. McLeod (2011) conducted the most comprehensive meta-analysis to date examining the link between the quality of therapeutic rapport and treatment improvement in child psychotherapy outcome studies. His results showed only a small association between the two variables ($r = .14$), suggesting that the quality of the therapeutic rapport had little impact on the degree of treatment progress. The implication of this research is that the impact of therapeutic rapport on treatment outcome with children may be much smaller than many clinicians believe.

However, therapeutic rapport is still an important factor to consider in the delivery of mental health treatment, including EBTs. If one is to effectively deliver treatment, the client must be agreeable to attending sessions on a consistent basis with the clinician; the client must be willing to implement changes or attempt exercises directed by the clinician; and, with many treatments, the client must be amenable to discussing memories that may prompt feelings of anxiety, shame, or guilt. All of these aspects of treatment can be aided by a supportive therapeutic relationship. In fact, some research suggests that a poor therapeutic rapport is a primary cause for early treatment termination (Garcia & Weisz, 2002).

Despite concerns from some clinicians that the use of treatment manuals and EBTs may impair therapeutic rapport (Nelson, Steele, & Mize, 2006), a recent study found that clinicians using trauma-focused cognitive-behavioral therapy (TF-CBT), an EBT, received comparable child-reported ratings of rapport quality as those clinicians providing usual care (Armstrong & Allen, 2013). Interestingly, caregivers with TF-CBT clinicians reported greater therapeutic rapport than caregivers receiving treatment from usual care clinicians. Further illustrating the point is a recently published clinical trial wherein adolescents with posttraumatic stress were randomly assigned to receive TF-CBT or standard community treatment (Ormhaug, Jensen, Wentzel-Larsen, & Shirk, 2014). Results indicated that the quality of therapeutic rapport was comparable across treatment conditions, but TF-CBT yielded better treatment outcomes than standard community treatment. In addition, TF-CBT outcomes were enhanced by a better quality of therapeutic rapport, and clients were discharged in fewer sessions. These results suggest that a trauma-focused EBT, such as TF-CBT, does not impair the development of therapeutic rapport, and a quality therapeutic rapport may improve the effectiveness and efficiency of an EBT.

Within the context of EBTs, therapeutic rapport is valued; however, it is not considered sufficient for change. Rather, quality therapeutic rapport is considered an important treatment consideration that increases the likelihood of successful implementation of the prescribed treatment techniques. Indeed, treatment manuals for EBTs often provide discussions about the importance of therapeutic rapport near the beginning of the manual (e.g., Cohen, Mannarino, & Deblinger, 2006; Kendall & Hedtke, 2006). However, EBTs do not typically consider establishing and cultivating a therapeutic rapport as the primary or only treatment technique. Instead, the specific treatment techniques specified within the treatment manual are considered the primary psychotherapeutic agents of change.

Treatment Techniques

There are many theoretical orientations within the mental health field (e.g., behavioral, psychodynamic, humanistic), and each one defines a theory of psychopathology, or conceptualization of why a particular emotional or behavioral problem develops. These theories of etiology lead directly to ideas about the types of experiences the client needs to improve and the techniques that a clinician should employ to provide the needed experiences (Prochaska & Norcross, 2009).

One of the requirements for an intervention to be designated as an EBT is that the treatment be derived from a sound theoretical basis. Although there are numerous theories that explain the development of a particular problem, not all theoretical explanations are supported by the empirical literature. As an example, consider the popular belief that bullies and other aggressive people tend to have low self-esteem and that their hostile behavior allows them to feel better about themselves. A considerable amount of empirical research suggests that people with low self-esteem do *not* tend to display aggression, and bullies typically report having *above average* self-esteem (e.g., Allen, 2011; Baumeister, Bushman, & Campbell, 2000; Thomaes, Bushman, Stegge, & Olthof, 2008). As such, interventions attempting to treat aggressive children by boosting self-esteem do not appear to rest on a sound theoretical basis, and it is unlikely that the techniques employed are effective.

Even with an empirically justifiable theoretical basis, the specified techniques themselves may or may not lead to therapeutic change. The specification of these techniques often is an iterative process wherein the results of previous research prompt revision of the techniques, which are then tested in future studies. Developing and testing complete treatment protocols and specific individual techniques utilize various methodologies; the process of developing an EBT is considered next.

TESTING AND VALIDATING PSYCHOLOGICAL TREATMENTS

Defining and testing an intervention to the point that sufficient evidence is available to designate it as "evidence based" takes considerable time, funding, and effort. In addition, the very suggestion that mental health treatments should undergo such rigorous evaluation and be graded based on the quality and quantity of scientific evidence is a relatively new development. Nonetheless, it is likely that any legitimate EBT has undergone a lengthy development process and that numerous methods of empirically examining the effect of the intervention were employed. Each method of empirical evaluation possesses specific strengths and weaknesses.

Case Studies

A *case study* is an in-depth examination of the delivery of treatment with a specific client. Detailed descriptions of the implementation of techniques and the client's responses are often provided as a way of demonstrating how other clinicians might use the techniques in their own practice. Clinicians of all theoretical persuasions report valuing case studies and view them as critical during the process of treatment planning (Allen & Armstrong, 2014). Many times a case study is the starting point as a clinician begins to develop ideas about what techniques appear most effective, and how to utilize those techniques, through the process of treating clients. Sometimes case studies serve as an invaluable tool for treatment dissemination as they can demonstrate how a seemingly routinized and predefined treatment package can be used with clients of different cultures and characteristics, how barriers to treatment implementation can be overcome, and how to apply the techniques to different presenting concerns.

Case studies require relatively little cost and time and can provide rich clinical information; however, case studies cannot demonstrate that the techniques themselves were influential in treatment progress. The mental health field has a long history of clinicians attempting to demonstrate the effectiveness of a particular treatment approach by providing a series of case studies. Often these clinicians use their own judgment to evaluate treatment outcome and postulate that the techniques were responsible for the seeming improvement. Rarely do case studies include features that would improve the quality of inferences, such as using valid and reliable assessment instruments and assessing multiple domains of functioning (Kazdin, 1981). Even if these more rigorous standards are employed, the very nature of the method prevents one from determining how much of the noted treatment progress, if any, was due to the treatment techniques and how much progress was due to other influences (i.e., client factors, extratherapeutic events, placebo/expectancy effects, therapeutic rapport). In addition, single cases cannot demonstrate the generalizability of the techniques beyond the specific client(s) discussed.

Open, Non-Controlled Trials

After specification of the intervention protocol, the next step is evaluating the effectiveness of the treatment on a larger scale. Clinical trials typically involve implementing the intervention with a group of individuals who present with a common problem or set of problems. An *open, non-controlled trial* does not involve a control group; all participants receive the target intervention, and efforts are taken to ensure that the protocol is delivered to each participant with fidelity. Although the number of participants in the trial may vary, it is not uncommon for open, non-controlled trials to enroll a total sample of 15–30 participants. The goal of these pilot trials is to examine the feasibility of the protocol and collect preliminary data on the effectiveness of the intervention (Rounsaville, Carroll, & Onken, 2001). These designs are well suited to identifying any challenges or barriers that might arise across participants, which might indicate a problem with the protocol and in soliciting feedback from participants about their experiences in the study. In addition, these trials can provide initial impressions regarding the generalizability of the protocol to more diverse populations.

An open, non-controlled trial is more cost and time intensive than case studies, but does not tend to be prohibitively expensive or demanding. However, like case studies, an open, non-controlled trial does not allow the unique contribution of the treatment techniques to be parceled out from the other factors that affect treatment outcome. Although positive results of an open, non-controlled trial do not validate the treatment techniques, these designs are often an important part of the treatment development process because the information obtained can assist in the design and implementation of a randomized controlled trial.

Randomized Controlled Trials

A *randomized controlled trial* (RCT) includes two primary factors: (1) there are at least two groups of participants, one receiving the intervention under examination and another not receiving that intervention (i.e., a control group), and (2) participants are randomly assigned to the groups. The purpose of random assignment is to attempt to distribute the impact of client variables and extratherapeutic events equally across the two groups. Because it is often difficult to predict how these factors will affect treatment outcome, randomly distributing them across the two groups serves to negate their influence by assuming that they affect both groups equally. For instance, random assignment typically results in roughly equal gender and ethnic distributions across groups. Theoretically, other client-specific factors (e.g., coping skills, intelligence, trauma history) are equally distributed as well. The result of random assignment is that treatment differences observed between the groups are not attributable to client variables and extratherapeutic events, removing this factor as a possible explanation for why the group receiving the intervention under examination performed better or worse than the control group.

Wait-List Control Group

Historically, wait lists were widely used as a form of control group for RCTs. In this approach, a number of participants receive the intervention of interest and a second group of participants receive no treatment. This second group is considered to be on a "wait list" and will receive the intervention after the first group completes treatment. The RCT typically concludes when the first group completes treatment, and the researchers determine whether the treated group achieved gains not observed in the wait-list group. Because both groups include client variables and extratherapeutic events as possible sources of change, finding superiority of the treatment group over the control group suggests that providing the treatment was the cause of the observed greater improvement. However, because the treatment group received three different potential sources of improvement not experienced by the control group (placebo/expectancy effects, therapeutic rapport, and treatment techniques), it is not possible to conclude from a wait-list RCT that the treatment techniques were effective and responsible for the greater improvement.

Wait-list control groups offer a relatively inexpensive way of testing an intervention in an RCT. Because not all participants receive treatment, fewer clinicians are required to complete the trial. In addition, wait-lists may already exist in general community settings because of understaffing, creating a natural opportunity to compare an active intervention to a wait-list control group. However, ethical concerns are raised about the use of a wait list as a designated and predefined control group to test an intervention (Cohen, 2007). In short, the researchers are knowingly withholding assistance to people who need treatment. An alternative option using a different sort of control group (e.g., community controls, active controls) would address this ethical problem and increase the methodological rigor of the study. Given these considerations, wait-list control groups are being used less frequently in treatment outcome studies.

Community Control Group

Another type of control group for RCTs is a community control group, in which control group participants typically are referred to community providers for treatment. In this design, some participants receive the intervention under examination, and the other participants receive referral information or are assigned to various treatment providers available in the community. The use of a community control group is meant to imitate standard clinical practice. In the case of referrals, some children and caregivers will contact a provider and receive treatment, while others will not. During trials in which children and caregivers are directly assigned to community providers, the treatment will vary from clinician to clinician. Using a community control group removes ethical concerns about withholding treatment from participants and evaluates the intervention of interest against the standard care provided in the community.

Using community controls is fairly inexpensive, as researchers are only required to provide treatment for half of the total study sample; however, significant problems are associated with a community control group design. First, with the referral approach, a number of children in the control group typically will not receive treatment. This creates a control group in which some participants receive treatment and others do not. The result is that the group as a whole may perform worse than if all children received treatment. Second, when children are treated by a community clinician, the types of interventions received may vary widely. Many children may receive treatment that creates relatively little change, while other children may receive more effective treatment. In addition, some children might receive treatment similar to the intervention being tested, which can make it difficult to ascertain the true impact of the target intervention. When using community controls, researchers face considerable challenges in ascertaining the degree to which the tested techniques were responsible for any observed differences between the treatment group and the control group.

Active Control Group

Considered the "gold standard" of clinical research, an RCT with an active control group provides the strongest level of support for an intervention. In this design, the control group receives an intervention selected, or at least monitored, by the researchers. A widely used method is to provide the control group with nondirective supportive treatment. Younger children in this type of control group often receive child-centered, nondirective play therapy. A clinician allows the child to select the activities of sessions, provides a safe and supportive environment, and only makes comments that are designed to demonstrate empathy, support, and positive regard. When treating adolescents, the control intervention often resembles nondirective supportive counseling in which the clinician allows the adolescent to determine the topics of conversation and the clinician responds with reflective and empathic listening. Consequently, the control group receives all sources of potential change (i.e., client variables, extratherapeutic events, placebo/expectancy effects, and therapeutic relationship) with the exception of more specific treatment techniques. As a result, superior performance by the group receiving the intervention being tested suggests that the greater observed change must be attributable to the delivery of the defined techniques. Findings of comparable results between the two groups suggest that the techniques were not particularly helpful.

Another form of active control design involves providing the control group with an intervention already possessing sufficient support to be designated as an EBT. In this case, both groups receive an intervention designed to treat the identified problem. Comparable results between the two groups indicate that the experimental intervention achieves treatment gains similar to an intervention already demonstrated as effective, and provides significant support for the intervention being tested. However, poorer results for the target intervention do not necessarily mean that it is ineffective. Rather, it could mean that the intervention is simply not as effective as the previously established treatment, but may still be superior to rapport-focused treatment if tested against such an intervention in another trial.

Although an RCT with an active control group is the most methodologically rigorous clinical research design available, it too has drawbacks. First, these trials tend to be expensive and time consuming. The researchers must fund treatment for all participants, as well as consider the costs associated with training, supervising, and monitoring the clinicians in the use of multiple interventions. It is rare that such a trial can be successfully completed without designated funding (e.g., a grant from an external agency). Second, regardless of whether one uses a pure nondirective supportive therapy or a previously established EBT, neither reflects true clinical practice in the community. Relatively few community-based clinicians are trained to fidelity in the use of a given EBT, and clinicians who primarily utilize a nondirective supportive approach may integrate more empirically based techniques. This makes it difficult to establish in an RCT that the tested intervention will perform better than the treatment provided by any given clinician using a different approach. Even with these limitations, an RCT with an active control group provides the only effective avenue to demonstrate that the identified techniques are responsible for observed clinical progress.

The Importance of Replication

Even with a successful RCT utilizing an active control group, the possibility remains that the observed findings were obtained in error. Factors unique to the sample or specific to the clinicians utilized in the study (e.g., allegiance to a preferred theoretical approach, interpersonal skills) may have created the observed differences, and not the actual techniques. For these reasons, replicating the clinical trial with a different sample of participants is often required for designation of the treatment as an EBT. Some guidelines require that at least two different researchers demonstrate positive results of the intervention in order to minimize the impact of clinician-specific variables or self-interests influencing the results.

The standard of validating an intervention is necessarily high and includes a sound theoretical rationale, a manual specifying the techniques or protocol, and at least two RCTs demonstrating that the techniques themselves are responsible for clinical improvement. Completion of this process with positive results creates confidence among clinicians, policymakers, and the general public that the techniques being employed are effective in ameliorating the targeted presenting problems. However, concerns and objections to the wider utilization of EBTs remain, many of which reflect misunderstandings about EBTs or express concerns that are not validated by empirical research.

MISCONCEPTIONS OF EBTs

• *EBTs are developed in academic settings and are not effective in the "real world."* A common criticism of EBTs is derived from a belief that research performed in a controlled academic environment does not generalize to community settings. The logic typically emphasizes that studies focus on treating clients with one or two presenting problems, exclude complex and difficult-to-treat clients, and fail to simulate the daily pressures and complications of clinical work. These criticisms, however, often fail to distinguish between *efficacy trials* and *effectiveness trials.*

An *efficacy trial* is a treatment outcome study conducted within tightly controlled conditions, typically with multiple criteria for including and excluding potential participants. Efficacy trials often focus on treating only a specific presenting problem (e.g., posttraumatic stress, depression). Clients who demonstrate other significant presenting concerns may be excluded from the study. In addition, the clinicians in the study typically receive intensive training in the model, have sessions observed by study coordinators to ensure fidelity to the protocol, and receive corrective feedback if deviations from the protocol are noted. Under such tightly controlled conditions, the criticisms regarding the ability of treatment protocols to generalize to "real-world" settings are legitimate. However, such rigorous experimental conditions are required to test the intervention, particularly in the beginning phases of protocol development. If a clinical trial did not have such rigid conditions and the treatment was found ineffective, numerous explanations could account for the findings. It could be argued that the treatment was not delivered in a standardized way to each participant; the treatment is successful for some participants, but not for clients displaying significant comorbidity; or clinicians were not sufficiently trained and experienced. In other words, with less rigorous conditions, the ability to judge the impact of the intervention is significantly reduced.

An *effectiveness trial* is a treatment outcome study that typically occurs in a community setting, not an academic one, utilizes community clinicians, and includes much less stringent criteria for selecting participants. The primary goal of an effectiveness trial is to examine whether an intervention with positive results in efficacy trials can achieve positive results in general community settings. In contemporary research, effectiveness trials are considered critically important, and significant financial resources from grant-making agencies (e.g., National Institute of Mental Health) are earmarked for the purpose of completing effectiveness trials. With positive results in effectiveness trials, the criticism regarding "real-world" applicability is addressed.

As one might expect, effectiveness trials commonly yield smaller treatment effects for EBTs than do efficacy trials (Weisz, Ugueto, Cheron, & Herren, 2013); however, EBTs still tend to outperform treatment-as-usual services (Weisz, Jensen-Doss, & Hawley, 2006). Multiple examples of effectiveness trials are available in the child trauma literature, including community-based trials of parent–child interaction therapy (PCIT) with child welfare–referred families (Chaffin, Funderburk, Bard, Valle, & Gurwitch, 2011), child–parent psychotherapy (CPP) and TF-CBT with children in foster care (Weiner, Schneider, & Lyons, 2009), and Alternatives for Families: A Cognitive-Behavioral Therapy in a child protection center (Kolko, Iselin, & Gully, 2011). Further demonstrating the point, Ollendick and colleagues (Ollendick, Jarrett, Grills-Taquechel, Hovey, & Wolff, 2008) conducted a literature review of treatment outcome studies and found that client comorbidity was common in treatment research samples, and that comorbidity did not typically affect treatment outcome.

It is appropriate to require EBTs to demonstrate their applicability to the "real world," and criticisms about the applicability of research-based interventions in community settings are more valid when a specific protocol has not been evaluated in effectiveness trials. However, most EBTs, particularly those related to trauma-exposed children, have demonstrated the ability to produce positive results in community settings with complex cases. As such, the criticism that EBTs are too academic and are not relevant to "real-world" practice appears unwarranted.

- *All treatments achieve the same results, so identifying EBTs is unnecessary.* Smith and Glass (1977) conducted a seminal meta-analysis of the results of treatment outcome studies. They concluded that behavioral and nonbehavioral treatments resulted in comparable outcomes, leading many in the field to conclude that all treatment approaches are effective at achieving positive outcomes. These conclusions were controversial at the time; however, as clinical and research methods were refined, it became apparent that not all treatments yield similar outcomes.

From a contemporary perspective, the most significant flaw of the Smith and Glass meta-analysis and similar studies published in the years immediately afterward, is the emphasis placed on theoretical orientation. In these meta-analyses, studies were collapsed into categories based on the theoretical orientation of the treatment being tested and rarely considered the problem(s) being treated in the studies. This method obscures an important clinical question: what treatment is most effective for a client with a given problem or diagnosis? In the past 25 years, most meta-analyses and reviews have examined the treatment of a specific problem or set of problems, not broad theoretical orientations.

This altered emphasis has led to important advances and the identification of treatment protocols that perform significantly better than others in ameliorating a given problem. Presently, the belief that all treatments work equally well for a given problem or diagnosis is rarely advanced in academic settings and among policymakers. Clinicians are encouraged to seek training in EBTs that target the most common presenting concerns that one is to treat as opposed to searching for treatments from a specific theoretical orientation.

- *EBTs are not culturally sensitive.* A legitimate concern of any clinician is being culturally sensitive. Cultural awareness and sensitivity represent foundational tenets of clinical practice. Two primary approaches to implementing EBTs with various cultural groups are evident in the literature. The first approach is to apply the standard protocol with different cultural groups and examine the effectiveness and acceptability of the intervention. For instance, the standard version of SafeCare (Lutzker & Bigelow, 2002), an EBT applicable in cases of child neglect, received high ratings of cultural sensitivity and acceptability by a sample of American Indian parents, and outcomes were similar to those obtained by other cultural groups in the study (Chaffin, Bard, Bigfoot, & Maher, 2012). A recent meta-analysis examining outcome studies of trauma-focused cognitive-behavioral interventions, including 883 child participants, found that 61% of participants in the trials were ethnic minorities and that ethnicity did not moderate treatment outcome (Allen, Henderson, Johnson, Gharagozloo, & Oseni, 2012). These results demonstrate a common finding in research on the applicability of EBTs across cultures; similar results are typically obtained across cultural groups (Huey & Polo, 2008).

Nonetheless, it appears that ethnic minorities seek out mental health services at a lower rate than their white counterparts (Roberts, Gilman, Breslau, Breslau, & Koenen, 2011), and ethnic minorities are more likely to prematurely terminate treatment (Wierzbicki & Pekarik, 1993). Given these considerations, a second approach to implementing EBTs with diverse cultural groups is to modify certain components of the protocols or integrate cultural beliefs and practices as a means of increasing the acceptability of the interventions to various cultural groups. For instance, recommendations on modifying TF-CBT for use with individuals of Latino/Hispanic (de Arellano, Danielson, & Felton, 2012) and American Indian/Alaskan Native cultures (Bigfoot & Schmidt, 2012) are available. Clinical trials of culturally adapted EBTs tend to obtain results similar to those obtained using the standard protocol (Huey & Polo, 2008).

It is important to recognize that cultural sensitivity may be best achieved by having a culturally competent clinician providing treatment, regardless of the treatment approach employed. Indeed, most published policies and treatment guidelines related to cultural competence focus on the awareness, skills, and attitudes of the treating clinician (Whaley & Davis, 2007). It is impossible to provide cultural adaptations of EBTs for all cultural groups one may encounter in clinical practice; however, a culturally competent clinician can effectively implement an EBT with diverse clients. In other words, the clinician may be the most critical factor in determining whether an EBT is delivered in a culturally sensitive manner. Whaley and Davis (2007) and Hays (2009) provide excellent reviews and recommendations on integrating cultural competence and the use of EBTs.

• *EBTs do not value clinical experience and creativity.* Traditionally, the mental health field emphasized the role of clinical judgment and experience in deciding which interventions to implement and in evaluating the effectiveness of treatment. With the advent and expansion of EBTs, these tasks are primarily determined by the results of standardized assessment measures and scientific research, which many clinicians view as curtailing their clinical freedom. Not surprisingly, some clinicians view this development as misguided and believe that their clinical experience and creativity is being undervalued or disregarded.

In actuality, EBTs do value clinical experience and creativity, albeit in a different manner than that to which many clinicians are accustomed. Although specific techniques are prescribed by the EBT, the clinician must determine how to deliver those techniques in a manner that will be most effective for a given client. For instance, if a treatment protocol directs teaching a client affect regulation skills, the clinician must determine what specific activities will be most effective given the client's unique characteristics. There are countless ways of teaching affect regulation skills, and many clinicians are quite creative in finding effective ways to achieve that goal. Despite concerns from some clinicians that EBTs neglect clinical skill and experience, an EBT must be implemented by a skilled and knowledgeable clinician to be effective.

- **EBTs assume that everyone is the "mean" and do not recognize individual differences.** Some clinicians object to using EBTs on the premise that research-derived interventions do not recognize individual differences. Often this criticism is directed at using statistical procedures to examine mean differences between groups, leading to the assumption that these research methods examine the "average person" and fail to understand or recognize individual differences. The reasoning then follows that many clients do not resemble the mean of a particular treatment group and, therefore, EBTs are not applicable to these clients.

Two primary misunderstandings are evident in this reasoning. First, the criticized statistical procedures use not only mean scores, but also scores of variability within the groups (e.g., standard deviation, variance). The amount of variability within a group directly affects the likelihood that a statistical test will yield a significant finding. In essence, these statistical procedures evaluate a group of individuals against another group of individuals, not a group mean against another group mean. As a result, when positive results are found in clinical trials, it is more accurate to state that a group of individuals who receive a treatment demonstrate greater improvement than another group of individuals who do not. It is important to remember that descriptive statistics such as means and standard deviations are meant to describe the group as a whole, not to describe an "average person."

The second misunderstanding of this criticism is the assumption that the treatment protocol should be administered in an identical manner with each person. Clinical trials require that the protocol be delivered in a standardized way; "real-world" clinical practice does not. For instance, although a clinical trial of TF-CBT may only allow for one session of teaching relaxation skills, it is often the case in clinical practice that two or three sessions are devoted to teaching a client relaxation skills. These variations in the delivery of the treatment will depend on various client characteristics.

Even though flexibility is permitted in the delivery of an EBT, it remains important to use the treatment as it was developed. Significant deviations from the treatment protocol, such as clinicians inserting favored techniques that are not prescribed by the protocol or declining to implement techniques with which they are unfamiliar or uncomfortable, may delay treatment progress and/or weaken the treatment's effectiveness. For example, it appears that some clinicians decline to directly discuss and process a client's trauma history (Allen & Johnson, 2012), even though this direct processing and desensitization to one's traumatic memories are considered critically important pieces of trauma-focused treatment (Deblinger, Mannarino, Cohen, Runyon, & Steer, 2011). Clinicians are encouraged to practice what Kendall and colleagues (Kendall, Gosch, Fur, & Sood, 2008) refer to as "flexibility within fidelity," in which the clinician practices in a manner consistent with the defined treatment protocol, but tailors the interventions to the needs of a particular client.

A CAUTIONARY NOTE

Terms such as *evidence-based practice* and *evidence-based treatment* are not copyrighted or otherwise protected by any legal or professional standard. Clinicians, authors, presenters, and others are free to use these terms at their own discretion and evaluate for themselves what constitutes sufficient empirical evidence. It is not uncommon for individuals to describe the intervention(s) they are promoting as evidence based, even if the quality and/or quantity of the research supporting the approach is weak. In the current mental health marketplace, amid the increasing emphasis by policymakers that EBTs be disseminated and implemented, it is almost a necessity that a treatment promoter convince clinicians that an intervention possesses sufficient empirical support to be considered "evidence based." One must remember that results from various research methods constitute "evidence," but not all evidence can demonstrate that the techniques are effective. Ultimately, clinicians are responsible for the interventions they implement with clients, and they are encouraged to verify claims that a particular intervention is "evidence based" before investing the time and money required to complete training in the treatment. The following online resources are available to help clinicians evaluate the strength of empirical support for interventions:

- California Evidence-Based Clearinghouse for Child Welfare
  www.cebc4cw.org
- Effective Child Therapy, sponsored by the Society of Clinical Child and Adolescent Psychology (Division 53 of the American Psychological Association)
  www.effectivechildtherapy.com
- Office of Juvenile Justice and Delinquency Programs (OJJDP), Model Programs Guide
  www.ojjdp.gov/mpg
- Substance Abuse and Mental Health Services Administration (SAMHSA), National Registry of Evidence-Based Programs and Practices (NREPP)
  www.nrepp.samhsa.gov

CONCLUSIONS

Developing, disseminating, and implementating EBTs significantly improves the quality of mental health care. The process involved in the development of an EBT is lengthy; however, demonstrating that therapeutic techniques are capable of creating change beyond the impact of client variables, extra-therapeutic events, expectancy/placebo effects, and therapeutic rapport is important in order to maximize the benefits of mental health treatment. The implementation of an EBT by a skilled clinician constitutes the best clinical care currently available for those we serve and should be the standard to which we aspire as a profession.

REFERENCES

Addis, M. E., & Cardemil, E. V. (2006). Psychotherapy manuals can improve outcomes. In J. C. Norcross, L. E. Beutler, & R. F. Levant (Eds.), *Evidence-based practices in mental health: Debate and dialogue on the fundamental questions*. Washington, DC: American Psychological Association.

Allen, B. (2011). Childhood psychological abuse and adult aggression: The mediating role of self-capacities. *Journal of Interpersonal Violence, 26*, 2093–2110.

Allen, B., & Armstrong, N. E. (2014). Burden of proof: The evidence clinicians require before implementing an intervention. *Child and Adolescent Mental Health, 19*, 52–56.

Allen, B., Gharagozloo, L., & Johnson, J. C. (2012). Clinician knowledge and utilization of empirically supported treatments for maltreated children. *Child Maltreatment, 17*, 11–21.

Allen, B., Henderson, C., Johnson, J. C., Gharagozloo, L., & Oseni, A. (November 2012). *A meta-analysis of trauma-focused cognitive-behavioral interventions for child and adolescent traumatic stress*. Paper presented at the annual meeting of the International Society for Traumatic Stress Studies, Los Angeles, CA.

Allen, B., & Johnson, J. C. (2012). Utilization and implementation of trauma-focused cognitive-behavioral therapy for the treatment of maltreated children. *Child Maltreatment, 17*, 80–85.

American Psychological Association, Presidential Task Force on Evidence-Based Practice. (2006). Evidence-based practice in psychology. *American Psychologist, 61*, 271–285.

Armstrong, N. E., & Allen, B. (July 2013). *The effectiveness of TF-CBT in community settings: Evaluation of an intensive training model.* Paper presented at the annual colloquium of the American Professional Society on the Abuse of Children, Las Vegas, NV.

Asay, T. P., & Lambert, M. J. (1999). The empirical case for the common factors in therapy: Quantitative findings. In M. A. Hubble, B. L. Duncan, & S. D. Miller (Eds.), *The heart and soul of change: What works in therapy.* Washington, DC: American Psychological Association.

Axline, V. (1969). *Play therapy.* New York: Ballantine.

Baker, T. B., McFall, R. M., & Shoham, V. (2008). Current status and future prospects of clinical psychology: Toward a scientifically principled approach to mental and behavioral health care. *Psychological Science in the Public Interest, 9*, 67–103.

Baumeister, R. F., Bushman, B. J., & Campbell, W. K. (2000). Self-esteem, narcissism, and aggression: Does violence result from low self-esteem or from threatened egotism. *Current Directions in Psychological Science, 9*, 26–29.

Bigfoot, D. S., & Schmidt, S. R. (2012). American Indian and Alaska Native children: Honoring children—Mending the circle. In J. A. Cohen, A. P. Mannarino, & E. Deblinger (Eds), *Trauma-focused CBT for children and adolescents: Treatment applications.* New York: Guilford Press.

Bratton, S. C., Ray, D., Rhine, T., & Jones, L. (2005). The efficacy of play therapy with children: A meta-analytic review of treatment outcomes. *Professional Psychology: Research and Practice, 36*, 376–390.

California Evidence-Based Clearinghouse for Child Welfare. (n.d.). Scientific rating scale. Retrieved June 14, 2013, from *www.cebc4cw.org/ratings/scientific-rating-scale.*

Chaffin, M., Bard, D., Bigfoot, D. S., & Maher, E. J. (2012). Is a structured, manualized, evidence-based treatment protocol culturally competent and equivalently effective among American Indian parents in child welfare? *Child Maltreatment, 17*, 242–252.

Chaffin, M., Funderburk, B., Bard, D., Valle, L. A., & Gurwitch, R. (2011). A combined motivation and parent–child interaction therapy package reduces child welfare recidivism in a randomized dismantling field trial. *Journal of Consulting and Clinical Psychology, 79*, 84–95.

Cohen, J. A. (2007). Ethical issues in designing treatment studies for traumatized children. In B. Allen (Chair), *Ethical issues in traumatic stress research with children.* Symposium conducted at the annual meeting of the International Society for Traumatic Stress Studies, Baltimore, MD.

Cohen, J. A., Mannarino, A. P., & Deblinger, E. (2006). *Treating trauma and traumatic grief in children and adolescents.* New York: Guilford Press.

de Arellano, M. A., Danielson, C. K., & Felton, J. W. (2012). Children of Latino descent: Culturally modified TF-CBT. In J. A. Cohen, A. P. Mannarino, & E. Deblinger (Eds.), *Trauma-focused CBT for children and adolescents: Treatment applications.* New York: Guilford Press.

Deblinger, E., Lippmann, J., & Steer, R. (1996). Sexually abused children suffering posttraumatic stress symptoms: Initial treatment outcome findings. *Child Maltreatment, 1*, 310–321.

Deblinger, E., Mannarino, A. P., Cohen, J. A., Runyon, M. K., & Steer, R. A. (2011).

Trauma-focused cognitive-behavioral therapy for children: Impact of the trauma narrative and treatment length. *Depression and Anxiety, 28,* 67–75.

Dowell, K. A., & Ogles, B. M. (2010). The effects of parent participation on child psychotherapy outcomes: A meta-analytic review. *Journal of Clinical Child and Adolescent Psychology, 39,* 151–162.

Garcia, J. A., & Weisz, J. R. (2002). When youth mental health care stops: Therapeutic relationship problems and other reasons for ending youth outpatient treatment. *Journal of Consulting and Clinical Psychology, 70,* 439–443.

Gibbs, L., & Gambrill, E. (2002). Evidence-based practice: Counterarguments to objections. *Research on Social Work Practice, 12,* 452–476.

Hays, P. A. (2009). Integrating evidence-based practice, cognitive-behavior therapy, and multicultural therapy: Ten steps for culturally competent practice. *Professional Psychology: Research and Practice, 40,* 354–360.

Huey, S. J., Jr., & Polo, A. J. (2008). Evidence-based psychosocial treatments for ethnic minority youth. *Journal of Clinical Child and Adolescent Psychology, 37,* 262–301.

Kazdin, A. E. (1981). Drawing valid inferences from case studies. *Journal of Consulting and Clinical Psychology, 49,* 183–192.

Kazdin, A. E. (2008). Evidence-based treatment and practice: New opportunities to bridge clinical research and practice, enhance the knowledge base, and improve patient care. *American Psychologist, 63,* 146–159.

Kendall, P. C., Gosch, E., Furr, J. M., & Sood, E. (2008). Flexibility within fidelity. *Journal of the American Academy of Child and Adolescent Psychiatry, 47,* 987–993.

Kendall, P. C., & Hedtke, K. A. (2006). *Cognitive-behavioral therapy for anxious children* (3rd ed.). Ardmore, PA: Workbook Publishing.

Kolko, D. J., Iselin, A.-M. R., & Gully, K. J. (2011). Evaluation of the sustainability and clinical outcome of Alternative for Families: A Cognitive-Behavioral Therapy (AF-CBT) in a child protection center. *Child Abuse and Neglect, 35,* 105–116.

Lewin, A. B., Peris, T. S., Bergman, R. L., McCracken, J. T., & Piacentini, J. (2011). The role of treatment expectancy in youth receiving exposure-based CBT for obsessive–compulsive disorder. *Behaviour Research and Therapy, 49,* 536–543.

Lutzker, J. R., & Bigelow, K. M. (2002). *Reducing child maltreatment: A guidebook for parent services.* New York: Guilford Press.

McLeod, B. D. (2011). Relation of the alliance with outcomes in youth psychotherapy: A meta-analysis. *Clinical Psychology Review, 31,* 603–616.

Mohaptra, S., Irving, H., Paglia-Boak, A., Wekerle, C., Adlaf, E., & Rehm, J. (2010). History of family involvement with child protective services as a risk factor for bullying in Ontario schools. *Child and Adolescent Mental Health, 15,* 157–163.

Nelson, T. D., Steele, R. G., & Mize, J. A. (2006). Practitioner attitudes toward evidence-based practice: Themes and challenges. *Administration and Policy in Mental Health and Mental Health Services Research, 33,* 398–409.

Nock, M. K., & Kazdin, A. E. (2001). Parent expectancies for child therapy: Assessment and relation to participation in treatment. *Journal of Child and Family Studies, 10,* 155–180.

Ollendick, T. H., Jarrett, M. A., Grills-Taquechel, A. E., Hovey, L. D., & Wolff, J. C. (2008). Comorbidity as a predictor and moderator of treatment outcome in youth with anxiety, affective, attention deficit/hyperactivity disorder, and oppositional/conduct disorders. *Clinical Psychology Review, 28,* 1447–1471.

Ormhaug, S. M., Jensen, T. K., Wentzel-Larsen, T., & Shirk, S. R. (2014). The therapeutic alliance in treatment of traumatized youth: Relation to outcome in a randomized clinical trial. *Journal of Consulting and Clinical Psychology, 82,* 52–64.

Prochaska, J. O., & Norcross, J. C. (2009). *Systems of psychotherapy: A transtheoretical analysis* (7th ed.). Belmont, CA: Cengage Learning.

Roberts, A. L., Gilman, S. E., Breslau, J., Breslau, N., & Koenen, K. C. (2011). Race/ethnic differences in exposure to traumatic events, development of post-traumatic stress disorder, and treatment-seeking for post-traumatic stress disorder in the United States. *Psychological Medicine, 41,* 71–83.

Rogers, C. R. (1957). The necessary and sufficient conditions of therapeutic personality change. *Journal of Consulting Psychology, 21,* 95–103.

Rounsaville, B. J., Carroll, K. M., & Onken, L. S. (2001). A stage model of behavioral therapies research: Getting started and moving on from stage I. *Clinical Psychology: Science and Practice, 8,* 133–142.

Saunders, B. E., Berliner, L., & Hanson, R. F. (2004). *Child sexual and physical abuse: Guidelines for treatment.* Charleston, SC: National Crime Victims Research and Treatment Center.

Self-Brown, S., Whitaker, D., Berliner, L., & Kolko, D. (2012). Disseminating child maltreatment interventions: Research on implementing evidence-based programs. *Child Maltreatment, 17,* 5–10.

Shapiro, D. N., Kaplow, J. B., Amaya-Jackson, L., & Dodge, K. A. (2012). Behavioral markers of coping and psychiatric symptoms among sexually abused children. *Journal of Traumatic Stress, 25,* 157–163.

Silverman, W. K., & Hinshaw, S. P. (2008). The second special issue on evidence-based psychosocial treatments for children and adolescents: A 10-year update. *Journal of Clinical Child and Adolescent Psychology, 37,* 1–7.

Simon, V. A., Feiring, C., & Kobielski McElroy, S. (2010). Making meaning of traumatic events: Youths' strategies for processing childhood sexual abuse are associated with psychosocial adjustment. *Child Maltreatment, 15,* 229–241.

Smith, M. L., & Glass, G. V. (1977). Meta-analysis of psychotherapy outcome studies. *American Psychologist, 32,* 752–760.

Thomaes, S., Bushman, B. J., Stegge, H., & Olthof, T. (2008). Trumping shame by blasts of noise: Narcissism, self-esteem, shame, and aggression in young adolescents. *Child Development, 79,* 1792–1801.

Villodas, M. T., Litrownik, A. J., Thompson, R., Roesch, S. C., English, D. J., Dubowitz, H., et al. (2012). Changes in youth's experiences of child maltreatment across developmental periods in the LONGSCAN consortium. *Psychology of Violence, 2,* 325–338.

Weiner, D. A., Schneider, A., & Lyons, J. S. (2009). Evidence-based treatments for trauma among culturally diverse foster care youth: Treatment retention and outcomes. *Children and Youth Services Review, 31,* 1199–1205.

Weisz, J. R., Jensen-Doss, A., & Hawley, K. M. (2006). Evidence-based youth psychotherapies versus usual clinical care: A meta-analysis of direct comparisons. *American Psychologist, 61,* 671–689.

Weisz, J. R., Ugueto, A. M., Cheron, D. M., & Herren, J. (2013). Evidence-based youth psychotherapy in the mental health ecosystem. *Journal of Clinical Child and Adolescent Psychology, 42,* 274–286.

Whaley, A. L., & Davis, K. E. (2007). Cultural competence and evidence-based practice in mental health services: A complementary perspective. *American Psychologist, 62,* 563–574.

Wierzbicki, M., & Pekarik, G. (1993). A meta-analysis of psychotherapy dropout. *Professional Psychology: Research and Practice, 24,* 190–195.

Yancey, C. T., & Hansen, D. J. (2010). Relationship of personal, familial, and abuse-specific factors with outcome following childhood sexual abuse. *Aggression and Violent Behavior, 15,* 410–421.

2

The Role of Assessment in Evidence-Based Treatment with Trauma-Exposed Children

Jeffrey N. Wherry

A good assessment requires a skilled clinician who uses data for understanding a client's needs and planning treatment, much like a detective uses clues to solve a mystery. A good assessment should include some systematic assessment of common symptoms associated with trauma and should utilize items that together are reliable, valid, and normed. In many ways, the development of psychometrically sound measures of trauma-related symptoms lags behind the development of evidence-based treatments (EBTs) for trauma-exposed children. This is both good news and, potentially, bad news. The good news is that trauma-exposed children and their families are receiving EBTs in many settings. The potentially bad news is that children may be receiving inappropriate treatment.

Recently, Conradi, Wherry, and Kisiel (2011) concluded that some maltreated children may not display specific symptoms indicative of trauma and, therefore, may not be candidates for trauma-focused treatment. For instance, not all sexually abused children evidence symptoms of posttraumatic stress or trauma-related sequelae and thus do not need trauma-focused treatment. However, after years of multiple disciplines neglecting the impact of trauma, policymakers have become increasingly attentive to "trauma" and "trauma-informed care." Unfortunately, this newfound interest and current fervor of legislators may not always be tempered or informed by the need for empirically supported assessments that lead to appropriate treatment. Thus there is the danger that uninformed clinicians will implement trauma-focused treatments with children who do not display trauma-related symptoms.

Consistent with this argument, Wilson (2012) recommended that children and their families must be properly assessed as a key step in the delivery of EBTs to address trauma and abuse. However, Dorsey, Kerns, Trupin, Conover, and Berliner (2012) note that these skills are rarely taught in graduate training programs. This chapter provides an overview of psychometric properties and their importance for selecting appropriate assessment measures, a discussion of the process of evidence-based assessment for trauma-exposed children, descriptions of reputable assessment measures, and how to connect assessment results to treatment planning.

UNDERSTANDING PSYCHOMETRIC CHARACTERISTICS

Many psychological tests are administered, scored, and interpreted almost exclusively by psychologists (e.g., projective techniques like the Rorschach Inkblot Test, cognitive tests like the Wechsler Intelligence Scale for Children). However, other instruments are utilized by nonpsychologist professionals with formal training in the ethical administration, scoring, and interpretation of psychological tests. Regardless of one's professional discipline, utilized tests should be psychometrically sound, which includes acceptable reliability and validity, and normed for use with the population with which it is used (Conradi et al., 2011).

Reliability

Reliability is the consistency of a measure, test, or tool (or its specific items). Reliability may include consistency across time (test–retest) or across independent raters (joint or interrater), as well as consistency within the measure itself (internal consistency). A measure and the items included on the measure should provide fairly consistent scores or findings across time and regardless of the professional who administers or scores it.

Validity

Validity is the degree of accuracy to which a measure, test, or tool (or its specific items) truly assesses the intended psychological construct, domain, or dimension of functioning. Various types of validity (e.g., face/construct, criterion/concurrent/predictive, content and convergent/divergent/discriminant) contribute to determining whether a measure is useful, meaningful, and truly measuring what it purports to measure.

Standardization of Norms

Standardization is the process of measuring a sufficient and representative sample along a psychological construct, domain, or dimension of functioning for purposes of characterizing a population. For a measure to be developmentally and culturally sensitive, the standardization should represent the population with which it will be used (e.g., by age, sex, and ethnicity/race). Collecting sufficient data from a representative sample is critical in order to place the results of the individual being assessed in the context of the greater population.

CONDUCTING A USEFUL ASSESSMENT

Assessment Methods

Historically, many different approaches were used when assessing children. However, Meyer et al. (2001) concluded that multiple studies document a high number of diagnostic errors when only one measurement or method was used. Generally, when feasible, it is best to use a multimethod approach. The strengths and weaknesses of different methods used to assess children are discussed next.

Rating Scales

Caregivers and teachers may complete *broadband rating scales* that assess multiple behaviors and symptoms (e.g., the Child Behavior Checklist). Other measures completed by adults (primarily parents) may be *unidimensional rating scales* assessing a single construct, such as depression, dissociation, or posttraumatic stress. Similarly, child self-report measures may be broadband or unidimensional in their design. These instruments provide an objective evaluation of the frequency and/or severity of various symptoms and can compare the obtained responses to other children of a similar age, gender, and/or clinical status. This allows the clinician to evaluate whether identified behaviors or emotions are significantly different from those generally observed from other children, or whether the concerns are developmentally normative.

If a unidimensional measure is used as the only instrument in an evaluation (e.g., a posttraumatic stress measure for a sexually abused child), it severely limits the breadth of symptoms assessed. When children (or adults) are presented with one unidimensional measure, they may use the presented items to force a description of the symptoms of concern. Not surprisingly, then, using a single unidimensional measure may result in a false positive for the symptom being measured. Alternatively, no significant concerns may be noted on the measure resulting in the false, uninformed conclusion that the child is exhibiting no concerns.

Using broadband scales protects against the problem of being too narrow in scope; however, broadband scales may neglect certain constructs of interest. For instance, the more prevalent broadband scales for children (e.g., Child Behavior Checklist, Behavior Assessment System for Children) were not developed to assess trauma-related sequelae (e.g., posttraumatic stress, dissociation). A good assessment should evaluate multiple types of emotional and behavioral areas (i.e., use of broadband measures), and incorporate measures to assess relevant trauma-related symptoms in a more focused manner.

Projective Tests

Projective tests are those in which children, theoretically, project their own psychology or personality into the drawing, story, or description of an ambiguous stimulus. These measures are rooted in the practice of psychology from as early as the 1930s and 1940s. While there is a rich tradition of using these approaches with children, their use remains more art than science. That is, the chief complaint related to these approaches is one of poor reliability in scoring (e.g., different clinicians may obtain different responses), as well as a lack of evidence for validity in interpretations (e.g., the meaning derived from responses is primarily a result of the clinician's judgment, not empirical research findings). Seldom do these measures have norms based on age, sex, or clinical versus nonclinical status.

Occasionally, a child may tell details of his or her story or refer to his or her experience while completing projective tasks. At times this information can be revealing. Rare responses occur with the use of projective tests that may suggest trauma status (e.g., a sexually abused child including genitalia on a drawing of a person); however, the available research demonstrates that even these more suggestive responses are not necessarily pathognomonic for trauma or abuse (Allen & Tussey, 2012). Some of these procedures (e.g., Draw-a-Person, Kinetic Family Drawing, House–Tree–Person drawings) may serve as a useful warm-up activity in the initial work with a child client, but clinicians should not overinterpret the responses or drawings.

One final mention is warranted regarding the Rorschach Inkblot Test—especially when administered, scored, and interpreted using the Exner Comprehensive System. While the Exner system is a significant improvement over past scoring systems, it remains a fairly complex and time-consuming procedure that may not directly assess dimensions or constructs that are helpful in understanding most trauma-exposed children. As with drawings, anatomically detailed dolls, and even rating scales, including suggestive responses to projective stimuli is not diagnostic for trauma or abuse exposure.

Clinical Interviews

The *clinical interview* (also known as the clinical intake, psychosocial interview, biopsychosocial interview) is the most often–used procedure by evaluators and therapists alike. The clinical interview allows the clinician to collect valuable information about the child's developmental and trauma history, the onset of presenting concerns, social support, and other relevant factors. However, even for a skilled and experienced clinician, it is possible that preconceived hypotheses are the only ones explored in this process. As a result, clinician-preferred diagnoses may be overidentified (e.g., a clinician primarily interested in trauma is prone to ask questions and interpret answers to support the conclusion of trauma-related problems), resulting in children and adolescents receiving inappropriate treatment. In addition, clinicians may fail to account for normal developmental behaviors and emotions. For example, a clinician assessing a 5-year-old trauma-exposed child may be inclined to view nightmares once or twice per week as indicative of posttraumatic stress, neglecting the fact that nightmares of this frequency is developmentally normative for a 5-year-old.

Some form of clinical interviewing, when used in conjunction with reliable, valid, and normed measures, can often elucidate descriptive findings. A variation of clinical interviewing is the *testing of limits* when using formal testing instruments. For example, when using a self-report measure, the clinician might administer the entire instrument and then score and interpret it as per the test's instructions. Then the evaluator might use the results as a launching point for interviewing the child, inquiring about examples of situations associated with the endorsed thoughts, feelings, or behaviors described by the instruments. A similar approach may be used with caregivers and caregiver rating scales.

Structured clinical interviews are procedures in which clinicians ask a prescribed series of questions, and responses are scored according to provided instructions. These procedures can help eliminate many of the clinician-specific biases that are involved with unstructured clinical interviews; however, these procedures are time consuming and may have components or modules with limited reliability and validity. In addition, using these procedures often results in high rates of comorbidity (i.e., multiple diagnoses made) with no process of differential diagnosis. This may result in overdiagnosis or misdiagnosis and, as a result, ill-informed treatment. *Semistructured interviews* allow more flexibility by the clinician while systematically moving through symptoms that are possible among children and adolescents. However, semi-structured interviews are fraught with the same shortcomings as structured clinical interviews.

Behavioral Observations

During *behavioral observations* the clinician attempts to observe the child and/or parent–child relationship in as unobtrusive a manner as possible. These observations can provide a clearer picture regarding the child's behaviors, interactions between the parent and child, the parent's discipline skills, and other useful pieces of information. However, like all other forms of assessment, the observations are only a picture in time and/or place, and may not represent the behavior of the parent and/or child in other situations or at other times.

When overt, externalizing behaviors (e.g., defiance, aggression) are identified in a home, classroom, or office, one may be able to hypothesize and test the role of various stimuli or events in the possible establishment or maintenance of behaviors using behavioral observations. For some trauma-exposed children, these observations may provide clues to stimuli or triggers that elicit otherwise inexplicable behavior by the child. For example, a certain tone of voice, a familiar look from an adult, or another sensory experience (e.g., smell or taste) may serve as a reminder of past trauma or abuse and result in a response that cannot be explained by the otherwise seemingly innocuous situation.

Multiple Informants

At its best, a good assessment of a child is a "snapshot" in time. Even when assessment results are integrated with history and findings from previous reports, they remain only a partial understanding or description acquired at one moment in time. To enhance the quality of the data used in an assessment and to increase the likelihood of providing appropriate treatment recommendations, information should come from several sources.

Caregiver Ratings

Parents and/or caregivers who know the child can be helpful informants as they spend the most amount of time with the child. Caregiver reports are vital for assessing concerns such as aggression and defiance, as children often deny having such concerns or may try to justify these behaviors. In addition, many clinical conditions (e.g., depression, anxiety) manifest external signs that caregivers observe and that children may not report.

However, these ratings of behavior from adults, like any assessment procedure, have potential flaws. For example, physically abusive parents may exaggerate reports of the child's externalizing behavior (e.g., defiance, aggression) that they believe prompted the physical abuse. Alternatively, parents who themselves are under significant distress may have difficulty with even minor behavioral problems and report significant concerns from a relatively asymptomatic child. Similarly, foster caregivers or residential workers can be influenced in ways that under- or overestimate the severity or frequency of problems. These well-intentioned caregivers may compare the child referred for assessment to other children who have lived in their home or unit and respond to items based on that comparison. Thus caregiver ratings, even when using instruments with outstanding psychometric qualities, have their drawbacks.

Self-Reports

For the child who is able to read with comprehension, self-report measures can be informative. They can provide information about the child's thought processes and emotional concerns, including important symptoms or concerns that caregivers are unable to observe. However, reading and comprehension alone may not be sufficient depending on the construct being assessed. For example, in the treatment of sexual abuse and physical abuse survivors, there often is a cognitive component to therapy. One of the goals of the cognitive component is to examine and often modify negative attributions that result in shame, guilt, and responsibility. Some children, depending on their developmental status, may not have the metacognitive ability (i.e., the ability to think about their thinking) to accurately answer questions about this process or their understanding of the trauma. A lack of sufficient metacognitive ability may make it difficult for some children to complete self-report instruments. This is a primary reason that self-report measures are not typically available for children under 6 or 7 years of age.

Teacher Ratings

Teachers can be another useful source of information. Positively, teachers are usually not comparing the child being evaluated to their best biological child or even their best or worst student in class. In addition, teachers are not typically directly involved in the treatment process and can provide a useful "neutral" perspective on the emotions and behaviors observed. However, anecdotally, it may be true that teachers do see behavior through an educational lens where such things as inattention and distractibility, along with defiance, interfere in obvious ways with academic assignments and with the ability to get along with others. Symptoms often described as internalizing (e.g., symptoms of anxiety and depression) may receive less attention. Occasionally, whether a child is referred by an agency or by a parent, the adults may wish to keep the information that the child was exposed to traumatic or abusive events confidential. This may negate the possibility of teacher ratings altogether.

Lack of Agreement

In any event, ratings and self-reports may show little agreement. For example, Rutter, Tizard, Yule, Graham, and Whitmore (1977) found that mothers and teachers agreed on the presence of behavior disorders in only 7% of children. Other studies have found similarly low agreement (Fergusson & Horwood, 1987, 1989), leading some to conclude that clinicians should expect some degree of disagreement among informants (Lee, Elliott, & Barbour, 1994). However, disagreements can provide useful clinical information. For instance, a parent report of significant behavioral problems in the home combined with a teacher report of a well-behaved child should alert the clinician to probable environmental factors prompting the concerns at home. Clinicians are encouraged to probe for the source of disagreements as a means of identifying potentially rich clinical information (De Los Reyes, 2011).

SELECTING AN ASSESSMENT MEASURE WITH TRAUMA-EXPOSED CHILDREN

Linking Assessment to Treatment

In identifying a useful approach to assessment, a good start is to use measures designed to assess symptoms that are common among trauma-exposed children. A variety of emotional and behavioral problems are common among children who experience trauma and abuse (Kendall-Tackett, Williams, & Finkelhor, 1993). Moreover, it is true that virtually any symptom imaginable can result from child trauma, although no single symptom is pathognomonic or diagnostic for trauma exposure. In cases of children who are exhibiting sexualized behavior, for instance, there are possible etiological explanations other than sexual abuse (e.g., exposure to sexually explicit materials on the Internet, observing parents' sexual behaviors at home).

Common symptoms among trauma-exposed children include anxiety, depression, anger, trauma-related symptoms (including posttraumatic stress and dissociation), and sexualized behavior. However, to assess only one of these dimensions alone is inadequate. Many children who do not display posttraumatic stress may exhibit other symptoms (e.g., depression, aggression, sexualized behavior). Some children who experience trauma may develop posttraumatic stress symptoms below the threshold required for the diagnosis of PTSD.

Different EBTs are useful for different presenting concerns, and it is important for clinicians to understand which EBTs are effective for which symptoms. With that knowledge, the results of assessment become invaluable tools for pointing clinicians in the most appropriate treatment direction. For instance, a child presenting with posttraumatic stress, depression, and/or anxiety following sexual abuse may best be served by receiving trauma-focused cognitive-behavioral therapy (TF-CBT); however, a child with significant defiance and aggression may be a better candidate for parent–child interaction therapy (PCIT), Alternative for Families: Cognitive-Behavioral Therapy (AF-CBT), or another intervention with a heavy focus on the development of parenting skills. Thus one of the greatest challenges in assessing trauma-exposed children involves both an accurate identification of the symptoms present and a concise conceptualization of the symptomatology, so that a coherent treatment plan might follow.

Evaluation of Multiple Symptoms Associated with Trauma Exposure

As described previously, broadband measures often neglect to measure trauma-related constructs (e.g., posttraumatic stress, dissociation, sexual concerns), and supplementing with unidimensional measures for each trauma-related domain may be overly cumbersome and time consuming. However, two notable measures that address this problem are the Trauma Symptom Checklist for Children (Briere, 1996) and the Trauma Symptom Checklist for Young Children (Briere, 2005).

Trauma Symptom Checklist for Children

The Trauma Symptom Checklist for Children (TSCC; Briere, 1996) is a self-report measure designed for use with children and adolescents ages 8 to 16. It is a 54-item instrument with two validity scales that examine underreporting (Underresponse) and overreporting of symptoms (Hyperresponse). Raw scores, T-scores, and percentile scores are reported for each of the following scales: Anxiety, Depression, Anger/Aggression, Posttraumatic Stress, Dissociation, and Sexual Concerns. As such, the TSCC provides an excellent picture of the child's self-reported emotional concerns, including trauma-specific constructs.

The internal consistency/reliability estimates for the clinical scales are generally considered good (alphas range from 0.77 to 0.89 in the standardization sample). Adequate convergent, discriminant, and predictive validity were demonstrated in clinical and nonclinical samples. The normative sample included 3,008 nonclinical children; 53% were female, and the racial distribution of the sample was 44% Caucasian, 27% black, and 22% Hispanic.

Trauma Symptom Checklist for Young Children

The Trauma Symptom Checklist for Young Children (TSCYC; Briere, 2005) is a 90-item, caregiver-report scale completed for children ages 3–12. It too utilizes two validity scales for the assessment of underreporting (Response Level) and overreporting of concerns (Atypical Response). Raw scores, T-scores, and percentile scores are reported for each of the following scales: Anxiety, Depression, Anger/Aggression, Posttraumatic Stress—Intrusion, Posttraumatic Stress—Avoidance, Posttraumatic Stress—Arousal, Posttraumatic Stress—Total, Dissociation, and Sexual Concerns. Use of the TSCYC provides numerous advantages. First, it is one of the few scales validated for use with children as young as 3 years of age. Second, it assesses numerous areas of trauma-related symptomatology. Finally, the validity scales allow the clinician to ascertain whether the caregiver's report might be skewed by factors other than the child's actual presentation.

During validation studies, the clinical scales demonstrated good internal consistency/reliability with alphas ranging from 0.81 to 0.93. In addition, scores on the TSCYC scales were associated with exposure to sexual abuse, physical abuse, and witnessing domestic violence. Subsequent studies demonstrated the convergent validity of the TSCYC with other reputable parent rating scales. The TSCYC was normed with a sample of 750 parents stratified to match U.S. Census data by region, parent educational level, age of the child, race, ethnicity, and child's sex.

The rate of agreement between TSCYC and the TSCC is reported as weak (Wherry, Graves, & Rhodes, 2008) to moderate (Lanktree et al., 2008), perhaps illustrating the lack of agreement often found between children and caregivers. These findings illustrate the need for a multi-informant approach to the assessment of trauma-exposed children.

Evaluation of Trauma-Related Constructs
Using Unidimensional Measures

When a measure like the TSCC or TSCYC indicates significantly elevated frequencies of trauma-related concerns, such as posttraumatic stress, sexual concerns, or dissociation, utilizing a unidimensional measure to understand more completely the nature of the problem may be valuable. Some of the more widely used unidimensional trauma-related measures are discussed below.

UCLA PTSD Index

Unidimensional measures for assessing PTSD in children are somewhat limited. Perhaps the most widely recognized measure is the UCLA PTSD Reaction Index for DSM-IV (Steinberg, Brymer, Decker, & Pynoos, 2004). Separate forms of the UCLA are available for completion by children, adolescents, and caregivers. The UCLA systematically assesses the frequency of each of the symptoms of PTSD identified in the DSM-IV, allowing the clinician to identify the most problematic symptoms. In addition, the UCLA includes a trauma history checklist that provides a more complete picture of trauma history than might otherwise be obtained. It is easy to administer and requires only a few minutes for completion. Internal consistency is excellent with a reported Cronbach's alpha of 0.90 for the full scale. Test–retest reliability is reported at .84 after a median number of 7 days. In addition, convergent validity is good, although to date there are no norms published for the instrument.

Child Sexual Behavior Inventory

The Child Sexual Behavior Inventory (CSBI; Friedrich, 1998) is a 38-item instrument completed by caregivers of children ages 2–12. The measure assesses the frequency of normative and unusual sexualized behavior in children. Studies indicate that it is reliable and valid, and scores are normed based on the age and sex of the child. However, there is no validity scale. Raw scores and T-scores are provided for three scales: Developmentally Related Sexual Behavior (DRSB), Sexual Abuse Specific Items (SASI), and the CSBI Total score. The DRSB includes behaviors that are not unusual for a specific developmental stage; however, an elevated score suggests an unusually high frequency of those behaviors. The SASI score includes items that are more frequently exhibited by sexually abused children. However, an elevation of the SASI scale does *not* indicate or prove that a child was sexually abused. Friedrich (1998) noted that these sexualized behaviors might be present owing to other family behavior, including watching movies with explicit sexual content, family nudity, or observing parents having sex.

Child Dissociative Checklist

The Child Dissociative Checklist (CDC; Putnam, Helmers, & Trickett, 1993) is a 20-item parent rating scale that assesses various types of dissociative behavior in children. Items are rated on a scale ranging from 0 (not true) to 2 (very true). These ratings are summed, and a cutoff score equal to or greater than 12 is considered clinically elevated, particularly in older children. The

CDC demonstrates acceptable test–retest reliability in samples of nonclinical and sexually abused children, and Putman and colleagues (1993) report good discriminant validity for the CDC.

Assessing Trauma History and Characteristics

A number of instruments, checklists, and interviews are available to screen for traumatic events. Various forms of child maltreatment and trauma often co-occur. Many times, the most concerning traumatic event or abusive experience for the child is not the one for which the child was identified or referred for treatment. As a result, obtaining a complete picture of a child's trauma history is an important assessment consideration.

As one considers the many assessment measures available, it is important to note that reliability and validity studies are difficult, if not impossible, to conduct with these measures. The endorsement of items by children or parents cannot be used as forensic evidence to establish that these events occurred. Rather, the value is for the clinician who is tasked with treating these children and families. One of the many instruments available for screening for traumatic events is the Traumatic Events Screening Inventory, which can be completed by the child and/or parent:

- Traumatic Events Screening Inventory—Self-Report—Revised (TESI-SRR; Ford, 2002a)
- Traumatic Events Screening Inventory—Parent Report—Revised (TESI-PRR; Ford, 2002b)

Unidimensional Measures for the Assessment of Anxiety and Depression

Many self-report and parent ratings can be used to assess anxiety and depression more thoroughly. These measures have value after children are first screened or assessed and evidence of these concerns is identified. A partial list of these measures is provided below.

ANXIETY

- Beck Anxiety Inventory—Youth (BAI-Y; Beck, Beck, Jolly, & Steer, 2005)
- Social Anxiety Scale for Children—Revised (LaGreca, 1999)
- Child Anxiety Sensitivity Index (CASI; Reiss, Peterson, Taylor, Schmidt, & Weems, 2008)

DEPRESSION

- Children's Depression Inventory–2 (CDI-2; Kovacs, 2010),
- Beck Depression Inventory—Youth (Beck et al., 2005)

Broadband Rating Scales

The primary benefit of utilizing a broadband measure is the ability to identify symptoms that might not be reported or detected by unidimensional
scales or those instruments assessing trauma-related symptomatology. Two
primary broadband rating scales are used to assess children and adolescents.
The Child Behavior Checklist (CBCL; Achenbach & Rescorla, 2001) is used
often in clinical settings, and the Behavior Assessment System for Children,
Second Edition (BASC-2; Reynolds & Kamphaus, 2004) is used more often in
school settings, although each works equally well in either setting. The CBCL
and BASC-2 are studied extensively and possess outstanding psychometric
qualities (reliability, validity, excellent normative samples).

Behavioral Observations and Coding

Observations and subsequent coding of child behavior can take a variety
of forms. For example, observations of parent–child interactions may occur
in settings that approximate some clinical analogue (e.g., free-play, parent-
directed-play, and parent-directed-chore analogues). Roberts (2001) provides
a thorough review of parent–child analogue observation protocols.

Other observations are made in natural group settings. For example,
the Direct Observation Form (DOF) is one part of the Achenbach System of
Empirically Based Assessment (ASEBA; McConaughy & Achenbach, 2009).
It is designed for recording and rating of observations of children ages 6–11
in classrooms, at recess, and/or in other settings. Raters can be paraprofes-
sionals like teachers or research assistants, although supervision by a quali-
fied professional is recommended. Interrater reliabilities for the DOF scales
are acceptable and range from .71 to .97. The Student Observation System of
the Behavior Assessment System for Children is another example of direct
observations made in natural group settings (Reynolds & Kamphaus, 2007).

Various treatment approaches used with trauma-exposed children
recommend specific observation and coding systems, primarily to assess
parent–child interactions. For example, in PCIT, the Dyadic Parent–Child
Interaction Coding System–IV (DPICS-IV; Eyberg, Nelson, Ginn, Bhuiyan, &
Boggs, 2013) is used to rate parental skill acquisition. A review of the DPICS-
IV is provided by Borrego, Klinkebiel, and Gibson (Chapter 9, this volume).
Lieberman and Van Horn (2008), in their description of Child–Parent Psy-
chotherapy, describe a parent–child interaction observation procedure that

combines structured tasks, free play, and a separation–reunion task. The procedure is based on the work of Crowell and Feldman (1989) and was modified by Zeanah and colleagues (1997). It provides an examination of how the child seeks and uses support from a parent in various circumstances.

Assessing Caregivers

A discussion of instruments designed to assess families and caregivers is warranted.

Child Abuse Potential Inventory

The Child Abuse Potential Inventory (CAPI; Milner, 1986) is a parent self-report measure used to identify those caregivers displaying characteristics linked to the commission of physical abuse. The CAPI demonstrates good internal and test–retest reliability. The scale correctly identified 96% of physically abusive parents, with the most discriminative items assessing distress, rigidity, and unhappiness. In addition, pretreatment scores predict the likelihood of further abuse among physically abusive parents in a treatment program (Chaffin & Valle, 2003).

Parenting Stress Index

The Parenting Stress Index (PSI; Abedin, 2012) assesses multiple types of stress encountered by caregivers raising children, including stress related to having a challenging child, problems in the parent–child relationship, and caregiver-specific stressors (e.g., health, relationship with spouse). Reliability and validity of the PSI is well established. The normative group included 534 parents of children, as well as 223 Spanish-speaking mothers.

Cultural Considerations

One of the basic requirements in assessment is standardization of norms utilizing a representative sample for sex, age, and race. Some instruments are not standardized, while others (e.g., the CSBI) were standardized on a sample that was primarily Caucasian. Standard interpretations of T-scores are appropriate when the family/child is among the racial or ethnic groups included in the sample. Unfortunately, for lesser represented cultures (i.e., non-Caucasian, non-African American, and non-Hispanic), the availability of appropriate, normed measures is scant.

Several principles of cultural competence deserve mention. First, the interpretation of any behavior or event should be neither ethnocentric (i.e., based on the majority cultural norm) or completely relative to the culture (i.e., cultural relativism). Second, there often is as much variability within a racial group as between racial groups. Thus it is important to learn about other cultures and practices related to child rearing, family structure, sex roles, religious beliefs, and levels of acculturation. Last, although much has been written about the potential advantages of matching clinicians with children by race, there has been little research regarding this issue with trauma-exposed children.

THE IMPACT OF ASSESSMENT ON THERAPEUTIC RAPPORT

One potential objection by therapists is the perceived interference with establishing a therapeutic alliance when the therapist must conduct an assessment with a standardized measure. Certainly, there are parents, especially in cases of child sexual abuse, who need sessions with the therapist to tell their story and to secure emotional support and direction from the therapist. Also, for some children, self-report measures requiring reading may seem too similar to a reading task from school. This may interfere with rapport-building for the child who has a long history of school and reading problems.

One potential solution is to complete the assessment after several sessions of rapport building and engagement. Another approach is to use one dedicated clinician for assessment. In this model, the initial appointment with the primary clinician is followed by an appointment with an intake specialist/evaluator who completes the assessment measures with the child (depending on age) and the caregiver. For instance, the child may complete the measures with the intake specialist/evaluator while the caregiver is in session with the primary clinician. Likewise, the caregiver can complete his or her measures while the child meets with the primary clinician or complete them at the next scheduled session.

CONCLUSIONS

Ultimately, a good evidence-based assessment can inform EBT just as a good imaging study (e.g., magnetic resonance imaging) informs a skilled surgeon. For now, the domain of reliable, valid, and normed instruments designed for the assessment of trauma-exposed children is limited, and there is increasing pressure from many sources to utilize screening questions and measures with no or limited reliability and validity. While checklists, "screenings," and algorithms may have some value in the assessment of children, the science of assessment, skillfully implemented by a trained clinician, likely will continue to play a key role in the complex work of understanding and treating symptoms in trauma-exposed children.

SUGGESTED RESOURCES

- National Child Traumatic Stress Network Measures Review Database (NCTSN), Measures Review Database
  www.nctsn.org/resources/online-research/measures-review

  Detailed reviews of many of the measures mentioned in this chapter, as well as others, can be found with a full description of psychometric properties, citations, reading level, and information on how to obtain the measures.

- California Evidence-Based Clearinghouse for Child Welfare (CEBC), Assessment Tools page
  www.cebc4cw.org/assessment-tools

  This site shares many of the characteristics of the NCTSN website.

- Academy on Violence and Abuse (AVA), Core Competencies:
  www.avahealth.org/resources/ava_publications/

  This publication reviews core competencies for training in trauma assessment.

ACKNOWLEDGMENTS

Portions of this work appear in Wherry, J. N., Briggs-King, E. C., & Hanson, R. (in press). Psychosocial assessment in child maltreatment. In R. M. Reece, R. F. Hanson, & J. Sargent (Eds.), *Treatment of Child Abuse: Common Ground for Mental Health, Medical and Legal Practitioners* (2nd ed.). Baltimore, MD: Johns Hopkins University Press. Copyright Johns Hopkins Univeristy.

REFERENCES

Abedin, R. R. (2012). *Parenting Stress Index* (4th ed.). Lutz, FL: Psychological Assessment Resources.

Achenbach, T. M., & Rescorla, L. A. (2001). *Manual for the ASEBA School-Age Forms and Profiles.* Burlington: University of Vermont, Research Center for Children, Youth, and Families.

Allen, B., & Tussey, C. M. (2012). Can projective drawings detect if a child experienced sexual or physical abuse?: A systematic review of the controlled research. *Trauma, Violence, and Abuse, 13*, 97–111.

Beck, J. S., Beck, A. T., Jolly, J. B., & Steer R. A. (2005). *The Beck Youth Inventories* (2nd ed.). San Antonio, TX: Psychological Corporation.

Briere, J. (1996). *The Trauma Symptom Checklist for Children*. Odessa, FL: Psychological Assessment Resources.

Briere, J. (2005). *The Trauma Symptom Checklist for Young Children*. Odessa, FL: Psychological Assessment Resources.

Chaffin, M., & Valle, L. A. (2003). Dynamic prediction characteristics of the Child Abuse Prevention Inventory. *Child Abuse and Neglect, 27*, 463–481.

Conradi, L., Wherry, J., & Kisiel, C. (2011). Linking child welfare and mental health using trauma-informed screening and assessment practices. *Child Welfare, 90*(6), 129–147.

Crowell, J. J., & Feldman, S. S. (1989). Assessment of mothers' working models of relationships: Some clinical implications. *Infant Mental Health Journal, 10*, 173–184.

De Los Reyes, A. (2011). More than measurement error: Discovering meaning behind informant discrepancies in clinical assessments of children and adolescents. *Journal of Clinical Child and Adolescent Psychology, 40*, 1–9.

Dorsey, S., Kerns, S. E., Trupin, E. W., Conover, K. L., & Berliner, L. (2012). Child welfare caseworkers as service brokers for youth in foster care: Findings from Project Focus. *Child Maltreatment, 17*(1), 22–31.

Eyberg, S., Nelson, M., Ginn, N.C., Bhuiyan, N., & Boggs, S. (2013). *Manual for the Dyadic Parent–Child Interaction Coding System: Comprehensive manual for research and training* (4th ed.). Retrieved September 30, 2013, from *www.pcit.org*.

Fergusson, D. M., & Horwood, L. J. (1987). The trait and method components of ratings of conduct disorder—Part I, Maternal and teacher evaluations of conduct disorder in young children. *Journal of Child Psychology, Psychiatry and Allied Disciplines, 28*, 249–260.

Fergusson, D. M., & Horwood, L. J. (1989). Estimation of method and trait variance in ratings of conduct disorder. *Journal of Child Psychology, Psychiatry and Allied Disciplines, 30*, 365–378.

Ford, J. (2002a). *Traumatic Events Screening Inventory—Self Report Revised (TESI)*. Unpublished manuscript, University of Connecticut.

Ford, J. (2002b). *Traumatic Events Screening Inventory—Parent Report Revised (TESI)*. Unpublished manuscript, University of Connecticut.

Friedrich, W. N. (1998). *The Child Sexual Behavior Inventory professional manual*. Odessa, FL: Psychological Assessment Resources.

Kendall-Tackett, K. A., Williams, L. M., & Finkelhor, D. (1993). Impact of sexual abuse on children: A review and synthesis of recent empirical studies. *Psychological Bulletin, 113*, 164–180.

Kovacs, M. (2010). *The Child Depression Inventory professional manual* (2nd ed.). San Antonio, TX: Psychological Corporation.

La Greca, A. M. (1999). *Social anxiety scales for children and adolescents: Manual and instructions for the SASC, SASC-R, SAS-A (adolescents), and parent versions of the scales*. Miami, FL: University of Miami, Department of Psychology.

Lanktree, C. B., Gilbert, A. M., Briere, J., Taylor, N., Chen, K., Maida, C. A., et al. (2008). Multi-informant assessment of maltreated children: Convergent and discriminant validity of the TSCC and TSCYC. *Child Abuse and Neglect, 32*, 621–625.

Lee, S. W., Elliott, J., & Barbour, J. D. (1994), A comparison of cross-informant behavior ratings in school-based diagnosis. *Behavioural Disorders, 19*, 87–97.

Lieberman, A. F., & Van Horn, P. (2008). *Psychotherapy with infants and young children: Repairing the effects of stress and trauma on early attachment*. New York: Guilford Press.

McConaughy, S., & Achenbach, T. M., & (2009). *Direct Observation Form for Ages 5–14 (DOF)*. Itasca, IL: Riverside.

Meyer, G., Finn, S., Eyde, L., Kay, G., Moreland, K., Dies, R., et al. (2001). Psychological testing and psychological assessment: A review of evidence and issues. *American Psychologist, 56*(2), 128–165.

Milner, J. B. (1986). *The Child Abuse Potential Inventory* (2nd ed.). Webster, NC: Psytec.

Putnam, F. W., Helmers, K., & Trickett, P. K. (1993). Development, reliability, and validity of a child dissociation scale. *Child Abuse and Neglect, 17,* 731–741.

Reiss, S., Peterson, R., Taylor, S., Schmidt, N., & Weems, C. F. (2008). Anxiety Sensitivity Index consolidated user manual: ASI, ASI-3, and CASI. Worthington, OH: IDS.

Reynolds, C. R., & Kamphaus, R. W. (2004). *Behavior Assessment System for Children* (2nd ed.). Circle Pines, MN: AGS.

Reynolds, C. R., & Kamphaus, R. W. (2007). *Behavior Assessment System for Children— Second Edition—Student Observation System (BASC-2-SOS)*. Minneapolis, MN: Pearson Assessments.

Roberts, M. W. (2001). Clinic observations of structured parent–child interaction designed to evaluate externalizing disorders. *Psychological Assessment, 13*(1), 46–58.

Rutter, M., Tizard, J., Yule, W., Graham, P., & Whitmore, K. (1977). Isle of Wight studies, 1964–1974. *Psychological Medicine, 6,* 313–332.

Steinberg, A. M., Brymer, M. J., Decker, K. B., & Pynoos, R. S. (2004). The University of California at Los Angeles Posttraumatic Stress Disorder Reaction Index. *Current Psychiatry Reports, 6,* 96–100.

Wherry, J. N., Graves, L., & Rhodes, H. (2008). The convergent validity of the Trauma Symptom Checklist for Young Children for a sample of sexually abused outpatients. *Journal of Child Sexual Abuse, 17,* 38–50.

Wilson, C. A. (2012). Special issue of Child Maltreatment on implementation: Some key developments in evidence-based models for the treatment of child maltreatment. *Child Maltreatment, 17,* 102–106

Zeanah, C. H., Boris, N. W., Heller, S. S., Hinshaw-Fuselier, S., Larrieu, J. A., Lewis, M., et al. (1997). Relationship assessment in infant mental health. *Infant Mental Health Journal, 18,* 182–197.

PART II

TRAUMA-FOCUSED COGNITIVE-BEHAVIORAL THERAPY (TF-CBT)

3

Trauma-Focused Cognitive-Behavioral Therapy

An Overview

Brian Allen and Natalie Armstrong Hoskowitz

Trauma-focused cognitive-behavioral therapy (TF-CBT) is the most recognized evidence-based treatment for children who have experienced abuse and trauma (Allen, Gharagozloo, & Johnson, 2012). The protocol was originally developed and tested in the early 1990s by Judith Cohen, Esther Deblinger, and Anthony Mannarino. As a result of convincing empirical support, TF-CBT is currently considered well established for the treatment of children with posttraumatic stress and associated symptomatology (Silverman et al., 2008). Although the original trials of the model focused on treating children who experienced sexual abuse, later trials documented the effectiveness of TF-CBT for children exposed to other traumatic events (e.g., intimate partner violence, terrorism, natural disasters). In addition, children between the ages of 3 and 18, from diverse cultural and ethnic backgrounds, are found to significantly benefit from TF-CBT.

THEORETICAL RATIONALE

As the name implies, TF-CBT primarily involves interventions derived from the cognitive and behavioral traditions. Within the behavioral realm,

47

significant empirical evidence supports the view that classical and operant learning are powerful etiological factors in the development and maintenance of posttraumatic stress (Cahill & Foa, 2007). Through classical conditioning processes, various stimuli, including physical reminders as well as memories of the trauma, come to elicit emotional responses such as fear or anger. To minimize the amount of distress experienced, individuals may attempt to avoid these reminders or memories. In some instances, these attempts at avoidance are successful, resulting in the temporary removal of distress, and thereby negatively reinforcing the avoidance; at other times these attempts are unsuccessful and significant emotional distress occurs.

To extinguish both of these responses (i.e., the emotional responses to reminders of the trauma and the tendency to use avoidance as a coping mechanism) TF-CBT places a strong emphasis on directly discussing and processing the traumatic event(s). The child is taught adaptive coping skills to replace the avoidance, reduce stress and physiological arousal, and to assist the process of gradual exposure to trauma reminders. Initially, this desensitization occurs through discussions of the child's memories, thoughts, and feelings, and later incorporates *in vivo* exposure exercises, which involve directly confronting physical reminders of the trauma. Additional behavioral techniques are used throughout TF-CBT to address other emotional and behavioral problems, such as teaching caregivers to utilize child management skills (e.g., praise, rewards, time-outs) for externalizing problems (e.g., aggression, defiance).

From a cognitive perspective, the primary etiological factor in the development of symptomatology is the presence of unhelpful thoughts. For instance, studies demonstrate that maladaptive cognitions, such as self-blame, may increase risk for various psychiatric concerns following childhood sexual or physical abuse (Feiring & Cleland, 2007; Valle & Silovsky, 2002). TF-CBT teaches children to examine their thoughts and how they influence their feelings and actions. Unhelpful thoughts, especially those associated with the child's trauma experience, are processed and restructured.

Although primarily cognitive-behavioral in nature, TF-CBT integrates components of other theoretical perspectives, including attachment, humanistic, and empowerment approaches (Cohen, Mannarino, & Deblinger, 2006). For instance, the influence of attachment theory is observed in the emphasis TF-CBT places on the involvement of a supportive caregiver, which may result in reductions in stress for the caregiver and improve outcomes for the child (Cohen & Mannarino, 2000; Deblinger, Mannarino, Cohen, & Steer, 2006). In addition, the humanistic focus on the clinician–child relationship is valued and viewed as foundational for the successful implementation of TF-CBT techniques (Cohen et al., 2006).

TREATMENT THEMES

Gradual Exposure

TF-CBT places a primary emphasis on the continual use of gradual exposure through direct discussions of the trauma during each session. Clinicians begin the treatment process by conducting a thorough trauma history and symptom assessment, and both the caregiver and the child are specifically asked about the child's traumatic experiences. The material presented in each treatment session (e.g., psychoeducation, relaxation skills) is directly connected to the child's trauma history and current distress. As such, each component of TF-CBT, not just the trauma narrative (as discussed later), is considered "trauma focused," and the clinician is encouraged to examine how each session furthers the goal of gradual exposure. For a more in-depth discussion of the role of gradual exposure in TF-CBT, see Deblinger, Cohen, and Mannarino (2012).

Therapeutic Rapport

TF-CBT emphasizes the importance of therapeutic rapport. Given that sessions require ongoing discussion of traumatic events and the corresponding likelihood of distressful emotions, clinicians are encouraged to attend to the quality of the therapeutic relationship with both the child and caregiver(s). TF-CBT clinicians should be genuine and adept at providing empathic responses and reflective listening. Indeed, recent empirical research supports the conclusion that a high-quality therapeutic rapport enhances the effectiveness of TF-CBT (Ormhaug, Jensen, Wentzel-Larsen, & Shirk, 2014). Although establishing a therapeutic rapport is critical for success, it is not considered sufficient, and clinicians must remember that gradual exposure begins at the point of the intake assessment. A goal during the initial sessions of TF-CBT is to set the tone for the rest of treatment; children and caregivers should feel comfortable with and trust the clinician while also understanding and expecting that treatment will focus on processing traumatic events.

Caregiver Involvement

TF-CBT is considered a family-focused intervention, wherein the primary caregiver(s) and/or other family members are encouraged to participate in treatment. Caregivers are involved during each session of treatment. Typically, the clinician meets with the caregivers during the last portion of each session to review the information and skills covered during the session with the child. Caregivers are encouraged to practice learned skills at home with the child and utilize behavior management techniques to reduce externalizing problems. In addition, throughout the course of treatment caregivers will be desensitized to the child's trauma and examine their own thoughts and feelings related to the child's experience. Caregiver involvement not only increases the effectiveness of individual techniques, but also gives the child the opportunity to share his or her experiences with a person who can provide emotional support long after treatment ends.

PROGRAM COMPONENTS AND CHARACTERISTICS

TF-CBT is a components-based model in which the clinician implements components in a sequential order. Although the specific techniques must accomplish the overall goal of the given component, how techniques are delivered depends on the clinician's judgment and the unique characteristics of the client. For instance, there are numerous ways to teach a child relaxation skills or provide psychoeducation, and the clinician must decide the most effective way to complete these components with each child and caregiver. TF-CBT treatment is considered complete after all treatment components are delivered. A typical course of TF-CBT treatment may last between 8 and 20 sessions; however, longer treatment lengths are common with more complex cases (Cohen, Mannarino, Kliethermes, & Murray, 2012).

TF-CBT components are summarized by the acronym PRACTICE (see Table 3.1). A detailed discussion of each of the components is beyond the scope of this chapter. The reader is encouraged to consult the treatment manual (Cohen et al., 2006) for in-depth discussions of each of the components and consult Cohen, Mannarino, and Deblinger (2012) for specific adaptations of the model for various populations and settings. The goal and process of each of the components are summarized below, and a brief discussion of special considerations is provided.

TABLE 3.1. Components of TF-CBT

P	Psychoeducation and Parenting skills training
R	Relaxation skills training
A	Affective identification and modulation training
C	Cognitive coping
T	Trauma narrative development and cognitive processing
I	In vivo exposure
C	Conjoint caregiver–child sessions
E	Enhance safety and future development

Psychoeducation

This first component of TF-CBT is designed to provide information about the particular symptoms and traumatic experiences of the child. This is typically accomplished with storybooks, handouts, or games and involves discussing the information provided by these sources, especially those pieces most relevant to the child's unique concerns and history. Psychoeducation serves numerous functions, including providing a relatively nonthreatening beginning to the gradual exposure process and normalizing the child's physical and emotional responses. With cases of sexual abuse, the clinician typically provides basic sex education so the child can use anatomically correct terms when discussing his or her experiences and become comfortable discussing sexual topics.

In addition, psychoeducation involves providing a treatment rationale for TF-CBT to the child and caregiver. The clinician explains the process of skill development and gradual exposure in a developmentally appropriate way to the child, as well as to the caregiver(s). Common approaches include discussing the clinician's own experiences using the model and providing a nontechnical review of the research base for the intervention (see Research Evidence for TF-CBT). The goal is to instill hope for improvement and confidence in the appropriateness and effectiveness of the treatment model.

Parenting Skills Training

Caregivers are taught to employ behavioral child management skills to address common behavioral problems, such as defiance, aggression, and tantrums. The clinician works with the caregiver to identify the potential function of the problematic behavior and implement appropriate behavioral interventions. Prominent among these skills is delivering positive consequences for desired behavior, perhaps through verbal praise and/or the use of a token economy system (e.g., sticker charts). Caregivers are encouraged to ignore tantrums and negative attention-seeking behavior and to utilize time-out sequences for noncompliant and aggressive behavior. For a more focused discussion of behavioral child management skills, the reader is referred to the discussion of parent–child interaction therapy (Borrego, Klinkebiel, & Gibson, Chapter 9, this volume) and to Cohen, Berliner, and Mannarino (2010).

Relaxation Skills Training

The clinician teaches the child various relaxation skills, typically including controlled breathing, progressive muscle relaxation, and guided imagery. Other relaxation skills, such as mindfulness, listening to relaxing music, and journaling, also are commonly used. The clinician should ascertain the child's and caregiver's current relaxation skills and incorporate them into the relaxation repertoire. The child and caregiver are encouraged to employ these skills on a consistent basis to reduce physiological arousal and to cope with various concerns at home or school. In addition, the clinician discusses the importance of using these skills to reduce reactions to trauma reminders as well as to cope with posttraumatic intrusive thoughts.

Affective Identification and Modulation Training

It is important for children to learn to effectively express their emotional states and identify when to use coping skills. Clinicians help children expand their vocabulary for words describing different feelings, including words that accurately describe their traumatic experience(s), and teach them to identify physiological cues associated with distressing emotions. This often includes demonstrating a simple rating system (i.e., Subjective Units of Distress [SUDs] scale) to help children differentiate the intensity of their feelings. Once these emotion identification skills are in place, the previously learned relaxation skills are discussed as ways of reducing the intensity of emotions. Additional coping skills may be taught to increase the number of techniques available to modulate emotions, including talking with a caregiver, problem-solving skills, and social skills. Understanding the impact of trauma reminders and intrusive memories on the child's emotions and encouraging the subsequent use of effective coping skills are key features of this component.

Cognitive Coping

The primary goals of cognitive coping are to demonstrate for the child and caregiver how altering their thoughts can reduce emotional distress and to prepare the child for the work of processing maladaptive cognitions related to his or her trauma. The clinician teaches the child and caregiver how their thoughts affect their feelings and subsequently influence their behavior (the "cognitive triangle"). The child and caregiver are shown how to evaluate their own thoughts through a process of weighing supporting and contradicting evidence to determine whether other cognitions may be more accurate or helpful and lead to different feelings. Practice exercises use concrete events not related to the trauma to refine and strengthen this skill. Caregivers and children are encouraged to practice at home and consider it as an additional coping skill.

Trauma Narrative Development and Cognitive Processing

A hallmark of TF-CBT is the development of a factual narrative of the child's traumatic experience(s). This narrative serves as a focused gradual exposure tool and allows for the specification of the child's thoughts and feelings related to various aspects of the trauma. The narrative itself may take many forms, such as being written as a book, a scripted puppet show, or drawn with captions describing the events in the pictures, among other media. Regardless of the format chosen by the child, it is vital that the narrative be an account of the child's memory of the trauma and that it be verbally described by the child. Posttraumatic avoidance at this point of treatment may increase for some children, and the clinician should be cautious not to reinforce the avoidance by allowing the child to circumvent verbally describing the trauma.

The development of the narrative typically occurs over the course of several sessions. At the beginning of each session, the narrative is reread as developed to that point. Thus the child becomes gradually desensitized through repeated exposure to their memories of the trauma. Throughout the narrative development, the clinician should be attuned to the child's verbal and nonverbal signals of distress, including having the child identify his or her emotions. When the distress level rises to a concerning level, the clinician can prompt the child to use the previously learned coping skills. Once the stress level decreases, the clinician should return the child to the work of developing the narrative. Ceasing construction of the narrative because of elevated distress may reinforce the child's avoidance of discussing the trauma.

Once the narrative is developed, the clinician and child should review it with a specific focus on processing maladaptive thoughts. This process incorporates the cognitive coping skills previously taught to the child. When a maladaptive thought is changed, the new thought and corresponding feelings are integrated into the narrative in place of the now discarded thoughts and feelings. Through this process, the narrative is molded into its final form.

During each session, the clinician shares the newly developed portions of the narrative alone with the child's caregiver. This allows the caregiver to undergo his or her own desensitization to the child's experiences and to process his or her own thoughts and feelings related to the trauma without being concerned that the child will observe the reactions. Children are often concerned about their caregivers' reactions, and seeing a caregiver struggle hearing the narrative may adversely affect the child's participation. The caregiver's own maladaptive cognitions can be processed as they arise. In addition, the clinician should discuss with the caregiver the upcoming conjoint caregiver–child sessions and how he or she can provide a supportive and accepting stance while the child shares the trauma narrative.

In Vivo Exposure

After completing the imaginal exposure process of the trauma narrative, the child confronts trauma reminders as they exist in the world. The clinician collaborates with the child and caregiver to identify places, objects, people, situations and/or other stimuli that elicit significant reactions and avoidance from the child. For example, the child may display a persistent fear of wearing clothes similar to those that he or she was wearing at the time of the trauma or may refuse to be left alone with a babysitter. Using the child's previously learned emotion identification and coping skills, a plan is developed that will assist the child in directly confronting and coping with the feared stimuli. The clinician must consider, however, that avoidance of some stimuli (e.g., the perpetrator) is adaptive and should not be confronted.

Conjoint Caregiver–Child Sessions

There are numerous times throughout the course of treatment when the child and caregiver attend sessions together. For instance, conjoint sessions may be helpful for learning behavior management skills or having the child teach the caregiver coping skills he or she learns in sessions. However, one of the most powerful interventions in TF-CBT is the conjoint session(s) during which the child shares his or her trauma narrative with the caregiver. As the child shares the narrative, the caregiver provides encouragement and acceptance and praises the child for his or her courage and work. The goal is for the child to end this component knowing that the caregiver is fully aware of his or her trauma experience, thoughts, and feelings, and remains accepting and supportive.

Enhance Safety and Future Development

TF-CBT typically ends by teaching the child and caregiver personal safety skills that aim to prevent future trauma experiences. The specific skills taught to the child will depend on his or her unique needs, but may include assertiveness skills, body safety skills, and developing safety plans. The clinician should not overlook the importance of teaching safety and abuse prevention skills to the caregivers as well. During this last portion of treatment, the clinician can help the child and caregiver plan for special dates and events, such as anniversaries of the trauma, birthdays, or developmental milestones (e.g., graduations, religious ceremonies), which may elicit upsetting feelings as they remind the family of the trauma.

A Phase-Based Approach

Treatment with TF-CBT is typically considered to consist of three distinct phases. The first phase of treatment (psychoeducation, parenting skills, relaxation skills, affective modulation, and cognitive coping) is designed to improve the child's emotional stability and control. The second phase of treatment includes the construction of the trauma narrative and cognitive processing, and represents the most focused effort toward desensitizing the child to his or her traumatic experiences. The final phase (*in vivo* exposure, conjoint caregiver–child sessions, enhance safety and development) is designed to consolidate treatment gains by demonstrating the child's mastery over real-world trauma reminders both in the present and the future. This final phase of treatment also includes issues related to treatment discharge.

Each phase of treatment is conceptualized as constituting approximately one-third of the total treatment time. However, anecdotal reports suggest that clinicians often remain in the first phase of treatment for an inordinate amount of time and may often fail to progress into the second phase. Indeed, a recent study found that, of the core TF-CBT components, clinicians self-reported being least likely to utilize the trauma narrative and cognitive processing components (Allen & Johnson, 2012). TF-CBT is designed as a sequential, unified model in which each component is important to achieving treatment goals. Clinicians are encouraged to implement the protocol as designed to maximize treatment effectiveness.

Applying TF-CBT in Diverse Situations

The component-based structure of TF-CBT lends itself to adaptation for diverse situations and considerations. For instance, in cases wherein the child experiences ongoing threats of additional traumas, the clinician may implement the "enhancing safety" component in earlier sessions and again as necessary throughout treatment (Cohen, Mannarino, & Murray, 2011). Other published recommendations discuss the use of TF-CBT with cases of "complex trauma" (Cohen, Mannarino, Kliethermes, et al., 2012), when substance abuse co-occurs with trauma symptoms (Cohen, Mannarino, Zhitova, & Capone, 2003), when children present with developmental disabilities (Grosso, 2012), and with children in foster care (Dorsey & Deblinger, 2012), among other considerations.

RESEARCH EVIDENCE FOR TF-CBT

A substantial body of empirical evidence examining TF-CBT is available. Randomized controlled trials demonstrate the superiority of TF-CBT over nondirective, child-centered treatment for the reduction of posttraumatic stress, depression, and anxiety (Cohen, Deblinger, Mannarino, & Steer, 2004; Cohen, Mannarino, & Iyengar, 2011), and a recent meta-analysis demonstrated effect sizes between small and medium in strength favoring TF-CBT over child-centered, rapport-focused treatment (Cary & McMillen, 2012). Follow-up studies document the maintenance of treatment gains after 1 year posttreatment (Cohen, Mannarino, & Knudsen, 2005; Deblinger et al., 2006), with one analysis showing treatment gains lasting for at least 2 years (Deblinger, Steer, & Lippman, 1999).

In addition to standard clinical trials, a number of studies examined the mechanisms of change that account for the significant benefit observed from TF-CBT treatment. These findings are subsequently discussed.

The Importance of Gradual Exposure

As mentioned previously, gradual exposure is a unifying theme throughout TF-CBT treatment. A recent dismantling study examined the benefit of TF-CBT when the trauma narrative component was included or removed for children who experienced sexual abuse (Deblinger, Mannarino, Cohen, Runyon, & Steer, 2011). Results indicated that children completing a trauma narrative displayed lower levels of fear related to the sexual abuse at posttreatment than those not completing the trauma narrative. In addition, results suggested that caregivers of children completing a trauma narrative displayed greater improvement in their own emotional responses to hearing about the child's abuse. It should be noted that considerable improvement also was evident in the groups not completing the trauma narrative, a finding that the researchers attribute at least partially to the gradual exposure inherent in the other TF-CBT components completed by these children. Treatment gains for all groups were either maintained, or continued improvement was observed 12 months after treatment completion (Mannarino, Cohen, Deblinger, Runyon, & Steer, 2012). These results suggest that many children will benefit from TF-CBT even if a focused trauma narrative is not completed; however, completion of the trauma narrative and corresponding cognitive processing may be especially important for children displaying significant posttraumatic avoidance and anxiety (Deblinger et al., 2011).

Altering Maladaptive Cognitions

One focus of TF-CBT is identifying and altering maladaptive cognitions related to one's experience of abuse or trauma. Evidence suggests that treatment with TF-CBT leads to significant positive changes in a number of cognitions, including trust in others, sense of credibility, and shame (Cohen et al., 2004). A recent community-based effectiveness study in Norway, employing mediational analyses, examined whether alterations in maladaptive cognitions accounted for the positive outcomes noted from TF-CBT (Jensen, Holt, & Ormhaug, 2012). The researchers found that TF-CBT resulted in more adaptive cognitions than treatment-as-usual, and these improvements were directly related to improved outcomes for posttraumatic stress and depression. Thus researchers concluded that a significant portion of the differences in treatment response between children receiving TF-CBT and those receiving community-based treatment-as-usual was attributable to improving maladaptive cognitions.

Caregiver Involvement

In addition to findings that TF-CBT significantly improves caregiver support for the child, greater confidence in one's parenting ability, and reductions in the abuse-related emotional distress of caregivers (Cohen et al., 2004), these improvements appear to enhance outcomes for the children (Cohen & Mannarino, 1996). Deblinger, Lippmann, and Steer (1996) conducted a clinical trial in which TF-CBT was provided under three different conditions: TF-CBT with the caregiver and child, TF-CBT with the child alone, or TF-CBT with the caregiver alone. Reductions in children's posttraumatic stress symptoms were noted for both conditions directly involving the child; however, decreases in children's behavioral problems and depressive symptoms were noted for both conditions involving the caregivers. During the dismantling study discussed previously (Deblinger et al., 2011), children and caregivers assigned to conditions not completing a trauma narrative received additional sessions devoted to developing caregiver behavior management skills. These groups displayed greater reductions in children's externalizing behavior problems than the groups that did complete a trauma narrative.

Collectively, the research on caregiver involvement demonstrates that TF-CBT treatment provides a number of benefits directly to caregiver participants. First, caregivers experience reductions in their own emotional distress related to their child's experience of abuse or trauma. Second, caregivers report greater levels of support for their child after completing TF-CBT. Last, caregivers learn effective child management skills and report greater confidence in their parenting abilities. Perhaps most important, the involvement of a caregiver in a child's TF-CBT treatment appears to exert a profound influence on the child's treatment progress. As a result of this research, TF-CBT developers strongly encourage the involvement of a supportive, nonoffending caregiver (e.g., biological parent, kin relationship, foster caregiver, residential treatment facility staff member) in the child's treatment (Cohen, Mannarino, & Navarro, 2012; Dorsey & Deblinger, 2012).

COST-EFFECTIVENESS OF TF-CBT

A common barrier to implementing any evidence-based treatment, including TF-CBT, is the cost associated with receiving training, consultation, and the loss of revenue incurred from the time required for training activities. A recent study by Greer, Grasso, Cohen, and Webb (2014) evaluated the cost effectiveness of implementing TF-CBT on a statewide scale. They compared a sample of 90 children who received TF-CBT from clinicians participating in an intensive TF-CBT training program to a sample of 90 children who did not receive TF-CBT. After controlling for age, gender, race, and other characteristics, the TF-CBT group exhibited average cost savings of approximately $1,700 per child from the time of admission to 1-year postadmission when compared to the treatment-as-usual group. In addition, children in the TF-CBT group were significantly less likely to use more intensive services such as inpatient hospitalization, day treatment, and wraparound services. The researchers concluded that the financial savings of employing and sustaining TF-CBT were significant and worth the initial cost required for training and implementation.

CULTURAL CONSIDERATIONS

Like other evidence-based treatments, TF-CBT should be delivered in a culturally sensitive and competent manner. Cohen et al. (2006) emphasize that clinicians should make a concerted effort to become educated about different cultures and incorporate that understanding into TF-CBT treatment. The TF-CBT model is flexible and allows the integration of cultural beliefs and practices. For example, specific adaptations of TF-CBT are currently available for two different cultural groups: Latino/Hispanic and Indian/Alaskan Native populations.

In modifying TF-CBT for Latino/Hispanic families (De Arellano, Danielson, & Felton, 2012), particular attention was given to how certain cultural constructs, such as *machismo, familismo,* and *personalismo,* influence the treatment process and delivery of treatment techniques. For example, clinicians should recognize the importance in Latino culture of maintaining close relationships with the family (*familismo*). Practice modifications might include incorporating extended family members, including grandparents, aunts, and uncles, into treatment and placing a special emphasis on improving family communication skills.

The TF-CBT modification for Indian/Alaskan Native (I/AN) cultures follows a circular structure akin to a Medicine Wheel, which is historically considered sacred to I/AN groups (Bigfoot & Schmidt, 2012). The core

PRACTICE components of TF-CBT are modified and adapted into the Medicine Wheel circle, and then employed during treatment. For example, the trauma narrative is adapted into a journey stick or traditional dance, as traditional I/AN ceremonies have incorporated gradual exposure exercises for many years.

The successful adaptation of TF-CBT for use with youth of various ethnic backgrounds is positive in several respects. First, it illustrates that TF-CBT is a flexible model and is acceptable to children and families from varying cultural backgrounds. Second, it highlights the practicality of incorporating culturally sensitive and competent practices into evidence-based treatment, a practice that may increase the likelihood of retention and treatment completion (Bigfoot & Schmidt, 2012; Cohen et al., 2006; De Arellano et al., 2012). Last, and perhaps most important, is the implication that TF-CBT can be effectively modified to assist clinicians working with other cultures in diverse areas of the world. For instance, Murray et al. (2013) discuss how cultural modifications to TF-CBT successfully reduced PTSD symptoms of children living in Zambia. Although it is not possible to develop specific adaptations of TF-CBT, or any intervention, for every culture, the successful adaptations for Latino/Hispanic, Indian/Alaskan Native, and Zambian cultures suggest that TF-CBT is a culturally sensitive intervention.

TRAINING PROGRAMS AND RESOURCES

A certification process that identifies clinicians who complete specified training criteria designed to establish proficiency in the use of the model (*http://rtfweb.wpahs.org/tfcbt*) is available . To qualify for certification, clinicians must have a minimum of a master's degree in a mental health discipline and be independently licensed to practice. Required specialized training in TF-CBT includes the completion of an online training program that provides didactic instruction in the components of the model (*http://tfcbt.musc.edu*), attendance at a live 2-day training conducted by an approved TF-CBT trainer, and participation on a requisite number of telephone consultation calls with the trainer. In addition, clinicians are required to complete three full TF-CBT protocols while using standardized assessment measures.

Training and consultation with approved TF-CBT trainers can be obtained through numerous state and federally funded training programs (e.g., state-level initiatives, the National Child Traumatic Stress Network), as well as through nonprofit organizations (e.g., children's advocacy center networks). In addition, training opportunities are frequently offered through collaboration with various professional societies and conferences. A free consultation website, containing answers, explanations, and demonstrations for commonly asked questions and clinical concerns, is also available (*http://www.musc.edu/tfcbtconsult*).

A NOTE ON TREATMENT PLANNING

TF-CBT is designed and effective for children displaying posttraumatic stress and associated symptomatology; however, anecdotal reports suggest that some clinicians may implement TF-CBT solely on the basis of a child's reported history of abuse or trauma. It appears that many clinicians are unaware of other available evidence-based treatments (Allen et al., 2012), and TF-CBT becomes the default intervention for any child with a trauma history. In instances where trauma-related problems are not a treatment consideration (e.g., posttraumatic stress, depression, trauma-related maladaptive cognitions), other evidence-based treatments may be more appropriate (Cohen et al., 2010). For instance, a child presenting with significant aggression and oppositional behavior may be better served by a focused parent training intervention, such as parent–child interaction therapy. Prior to beginning any treatment program, a thorough trauma-sensitive assessment using standardized measures should be completed and the most appropriate intervention selected based on the presenting symptoms and concerns (see Wherry, Chapter 2, this volume).

CONCLUSIONS

TF-CBT is an effective intervention for children experiencing posttraumatic stress, depression, anxiety, and other concerns related to the experience of abuse or trauma. The considerable empirical base for TF-CBT demonstrates the effectiveness of the protocol beyond the benefit that might be observed solely from nonspecific factors, such as the passage of time or therapeutic rapport. In addition, the flexible component-based nature of the treatment is amenable to various cultural and clinical considerations. Although TF-CBT is not a panacea, it should be a primary treatment modality for clinicians who serve trauma-exposed children.

SUGGESTED RESOURCES

Books

- Cohen, J. A., Mannarino, A. P., & Deblinger, E. (2006). *Treating trauma and traumatic grief in children and adolescents.* New York: Guilford Press.
- Cohen, J. A., Mannarino, A. P., & Deblinger, E. (Eds.). (2012). *Trauma-focused CBT for children and adolescents: Treatment applications.* New York: Guilford Press.

Websites

- TF-CBT*Web* (didactic training in the components of TF-CBT)
  http://tfcbt.musc.edu

- TF-CBT*Consult* (answers to frequently asked questions)
  http://www.musc.edu/tfcbtconsult

- Allegheny General Hospital Center for Traumatic Stress in Children and Adolescents
  www.wpahs.org/specialties/center-traumatic-stress-children-and-adolescents

- Rowan University Child Abuse Research, Education, & Service (CARES) Institute
  www.caresinstitute.org

REFERENCES

Allen, B., Gharagozloo, L., & Johnson, J. C. (2012). Clinician knowledge and utilization of empirically-supported treatments for maltreated children. *Child Maltreatment, 17*, 11–21.

Allen, B., & Johnson, J. C. (2012). Utilization and implementation of trauma-focused cognitive-behavioral therapy for the treatment of maltreated children. *Child Maltreatment, 17*, 80–85.

Bigfoot, D. S., & Schmidt, S. R. (2012). American Indian and Alaska Native children: Honoring children—Mending the circle. In J. A. Cohen, A. P. Mannarino, & E. Deblinger (Eds.), *Trauma-focused CBT for children and adolescents: Treatment applications*. New York: Guilford Press.

Cahill, S. P., & Foa, E. B. (2007). Psychological theories of PTSD. In M. J. Friedman, T. M. Keane, & P. A. Resick (Eds.), *Handbook of PTSD: Science and practice*. New York: Guilford Press.

Cary, C. E., & McMillen, J. C. (2012). The data behind the dissemination: A systematic review of trauma-focused cognitive-behavioral therapy for use with children and youth. *Children and Youth Services Review, 34*, 748–757.

Cohen, J. A., Berliner, L., & Mannarino, A. P. (2010). Trauma-focused CBT for children with co-occurring trauma and behavior problems. *Child Abuse and Neglect, 34*, 215–224.

Cohen, J. A., Deblinger, E., Mannarino, A. P., & Steer, R. A. (2004). A multisite, randomized controlled trial for children with sexual abuse-related PTSD symptoms. *Journal of the American Academy of Child and Adolescent Psychiatry, 43*, 393–402.

Cohen, J. A., & Mannarino, A. P. (1996). Factors that mediate treatment outcome of sexually abused preschool children. *Journal of the American Academy of Child and Adolescent Psychiatry, 35*, 1402–1410.

Cohen, J. A., & Mannarino, A. P. (2000). Predictors of treatment outcome in sexually abused children. *Child Abuse and Neglect, 24*, 983–994.

Cohen, J. A., Mannarino, A. P., & Deblinger, E. (2006). *Treating trauma and traumatic grief in children and adolescents*. New York: Guilford Press.

Cohen, J. A., Mannarino, A. P., & Deblinger, E. (Eds.). (2012). *Trauma-focused CBT for children and adolescents: Treatment applications*. New York: Guilford Press.

Cohen, J. A., Mannarino, A. P., & Iyengar, S. (2011). Community treatment of posttraumatic stress disorder for children exposed to intimate partner violence. *Archives of Pediatric and Adolescent Medicine, 165*, 16–21.

Cohen, J. A., Mannarino, A. P., Kliethermes, M., & Murray, L. A. (2012). Trauma-focused CBT for youth with complex trauma. *Child Abuse and Neglect, 36*, 528–541.

Cohen, J. A., Mannarino, A. P., & Knudsen, K. (2005). Treating sexually abused children: 1 year follow-up of a randomized controlled trial. *Child Abuse and Neglect, 29*, 135–145.

Cohen, J. A., Mannarino, A. P., & Murray, L. K. (2011). Trauma-focused CBT for youth who experience ongoing traumas. *Child Abuse and Neglect, 35*, 637–646.

Cohen, J. A., Mannarino, A. P., & Navarro, D. (2012). Residential treatment. In J. A. Cohen, A. P. Mannarino, & E. Deblinger (Eds.), *Trauma-focused CBT for children and adolescents: Treatment applications*. New York: Guilford Press.

Cohen, J. A., Mannarino, A. P., Zhitova, A. C., & Capone, M. E. (2003). Treating child abuse-related posttraumatic stress and comorbid substance abuse in adolescents. *Child Abuse and Neglect, 27*, 1345–1365.

De Arellano, M. A., Danielson, C. K., & Felton, J. W. (2012). Children of Latino descent: Culturally modified TF-CBT. In J. A. Cohen, A. P. Mannarino, & E. Deblinger (Eds.), *Trauma-focused CBT for children and adolescents: Treatment applications*. New York: Guilford Press.

Deblinger, E., Cohen, J. A., & Mannarino, A. P. (2012). Introduction. In J. A. Cohen, A. P. Mannarino, & E. Deblinger (Eds.), *Trauma-focused CBT for children and adolescents: Treatment applications*. New York: Guilford Press.

Deblinger, E., Lippmann, J., & Steer, R. A. (1996). Sexually abused children suffering posttraumatic stress symptoms: Initial treatment outcome findings. *Child Maltreatment, 1*, 310–321.

Deblinger, E., Mannarino, A. P., Cohen, J. A., Runyon, M. K., & Steer, R. A. (2011). Trauma-focused cognitive-behavioral therapy for children: Impact of the trauma narrative and treatment length. *Depression and Anxiety, 28*, 97–75.

Deblinger, E., Mannarino, A. P., Cohen, J. A., & Steer, R. A. (2006). A follow-up study of a multisite, randomized, controlled trial for children with sexual abuse-related PTSD symptoms. *Journal of the American Academy of Child and Adolescent Psychiatry, 45*, 1474–1484.

Deblinger, E., Steer, R. A., & Lippmann, J. (1999). Two-year follow-up study of cognitive-behavioral therapy for sexually abused children suffering post-traumatic stress symptoms. *Child Abuse and Neglect, 23*, 1371–1378.

Dorsey, S., & Deblinger, E. (2012). Children in foster care. In J. A. Cohen, A. P. Mannarino, & E. Deblinger (Eds.), *Trauma-focused CBT for children and adolescents: Treatment applications*. New York: Guilford Press.

Feiring, C., & Cleland, C. (2007). Childhood sexual abuse and abuse-specific attributions of blame over 6 years following discovery. *Child Abuse and Neglect, 31*, 1169–1186.

Greer, D., Grasso, D. G., Cohen, A., & Webb, C. (2014). Trauma-focused treatment in a state system of care: Is it worth the cost? *Administration and Policy in Mental Health and Mental Health Services Research, 41*, 317–323.

Grosso, C. A. (2012). Children with developmental disabilities. In J. A. Cohen, A. P. Mannarino, & E. Deblinger (Eds.), *Trauma-focused CBT for children and adolescents: Treatment applications*. New York: Guilford Press.

Jensen, T. K., Holt, T., & Ormhaug, S. M. (2012, November). Trauma-focused cognitive-behavioral therapy: The mediating role of negative trauma-related cognitions. In L. Berliner (Chair), *The application of TF-CBT in European countries: Scaling up evidence-based practice in child populations with PTSD.* Paper presented at the annual meeting of the International Society for Traumatic Stress Studies, Los Angeles, CA.

Mannarino, A. P., Cohen, J. A., Runyon, M. K., Deblinger, E., & Steer, R. A. (2012). Trauma-focused cognitive-behavioral therapy for children: Sustained impact of treatment 6 and 12 months later. *Child Maltreatment, 17,* 231–241.

Murray, L. K., Familiar, I., Skavenski, S., Jere, E., Cohen, J. A., Imasiku, M., et al. (2013). An evaluation of trauma-focused cognitive-behavioral therapy for children in Zambia. *Child Abuse and Neglect, 37,* 1175–1185.

Ormhaug, S. M., Jensen, T. K., Wentzel-Larsen, T., & Shirk, S. R. (2014). The therapeutic alliance in treatment of traumatized youth: Relation to outcome in a randomized clinical trial. *Journal of Consulting and Clinical Psychology, 82,* 52–64.

Silverman, W. K., Ortiz, C. D., Viswesvaran, C., Burns, B. J., Kolko, D. J., Putnam, F. W., et al. (2008). Evidence-based psychosocial treatments for children and adolescents exposed to traumatic events. *Journal of Clinical Child and Adolescent Psychology, 37,* 156–183.

Valle, L. A., & Silovsky, J. F. (2002). Attributions and adjustment following child sexual and physical abuse. *Child Maltreatment, 7,* 9–25.

4

TF-CBT with a School-Age Girl with a History of Severe and Prolonged Sexual Abuse

The Case of Mary T.

Clare Lucas

with commentary by Benjamin E. Saunders

BACKGROUND INFORMATION

Mary T. was a 7-year-old Caucasian female who received treatment at a child's advocacy center (CAC). Mary disclosed to a teacher that her adult cousin was sexually abusing her. During a forensic interview at the CAC, Mary reiterated her allegations of sexual abuse against the cousin, and the allegations were substantiated by child protective services (CPS). Her mother, Ms. S., requested that Mary receive mental health services through the CAC.

ASSESSMENT AND TREATMENT PLANNING

Mary presented as a quiet and anxious girl. She struggled to maintain eye contact throughout the initial intake session and spoke in a soft tone. She seemed acutely aware of noises in the office and surrounding areas, which was evident through her physically appearing startled when various noises occurred (e.g., a door shutting in a neighboring office, people talking in the hallway). The clinician repeatedly reassured Mary that she was safe in the office. The intake interview began by talking about general life events and her likes and dislikes, with the clinician constantly monitoring and attending to her anxious affect and behavior. The clinician believed it was important to address Mary's anxiety level in order to improve the quality of the assessment information obtained. Therefore, Mary was taught to use a simple controlled breathing technique to help her cope with her anxiety during the rest of the interview.

After learning and using the controlled breathing technique, Mary was more responsive to the assessment process and was able to answer questions about her traumatic experiences and current symptoms. The UCLA PTSD Reaction Index (Steinberg, Brymer, Decker, & Pynoos, 2004) was used to assess trauma history as well as symptoms related to the traumatic events. Mary endorsed experiencing sexual abuse, and her anxiety was noticeable when she began discussing the abuse. She reported struggling with intrusive thoughts and memories about the sexual abuse multiple times a day and would consciously attempt to avoid thinking about the memories. Many times her intrusive thoughts of the sexual abuse occurred while she was at school; sometimes resulting in episodes of enuresis that left her feeling embarrassed and teased by her peers. Mary discussed how any red car she saw would cause her to think about the sexual abuse as her cousin drove a red SUV, and that a polka-dot patterned skirt she owned would also trigger distressful memories because her cousin had asked her to wear it before some abuse episodes.

Mary reported being scared to fall asleep and lying in bed for "a long time" before falling to sleep. She would frequently wake up in the middle of the night from nightmares, and at other times would wake up experiencing a general sense of fear. The most distressing nightmares were about people dying or "being killed," and these nightmares occurred at least once per week. Mary was fearful of being left alone, especially at night. She described a fear that there were "ghosts in the house on the walls," and how she became scared when the ghosts were present. Mary also complained about headaches, stomachaches, and bedwetting. She did not like school and struggled with anger outbursts directed toward other children.

Mary became quiet and sad when asked about her relationship with her mother and stepfather. She worried about her mother's safety, especially during the day when her mother was home alone. Mary and her stepfather did not get along well, as they often fought and Mary was uncertain whether her stepfather even liked her. The only family members with whom she endorsed having a positive relationship were her younger brother and older sister. However, she was quick to point out her love for the family dogs and other animals in the home.

The majority of the background information collected was obtained through a clinical interview with Mary's mother, Ms. S. Mary's biological father was not present, as he lived in another state and had not been involved in her life since infancy. However, before he left the family, a number of physical altercations occurred between Mary's biological parents, and Mary was present for many of them. Most of the fights resulted in significant bruises and occasionally resulted in Ms. S. having a bloody nose. With the exception of the sexual abuse and domestic violence, Mary was not known to have experienced any other traumatic events.

The sexual abuse Mary experienced was ongoing for several years, typically occurred multiple times per week, and occasionally multiple times per day. Mary's adult cousin, who lived near the family's home, would often help baby-sit the children after school and on weekends. It was during these times that he would commit various sexual acts against Mary and require her to perform sexual acts on him.

More than a year before Mary began treatment, her mother began seeing changes. Mary became angry and had begun yelling at and hitting other children. At the same time, she displayed poor interpersonal boundaries as evidenced by her frequent touching of other people. Ms. S. noticed other changes as well. Mary had become more withdrawn and appeared at times to be "a sad and unhappy child." Mary worried constantly about her own personal safety, often looking out for anything around her that was potentially threatening. Mary's teachers were expressing concerns about her appearing to be "in her own world" and having significant difficulty focusing on tasks. In addition, her teachers had noticed Mary beginning to pinch herself at times and using "baby talk" when answering their questions.

Mary was diagnosed with posttraumatic stress disorder (PTSD). Because of the long-standing nature of Mary's PTSD symptoms the specifier of "chronic" was added to the diagnosis. Mary was also given a secondary diagnoses of major depressive disorder and generalized anxiety disorder.

Mary's history and symptoms suggested that the TF-CBT model would most likely provide the greatest benefit. The treating clinician (a licensed, master's-level counselor with previous training and experience using TF-CBT) provided Ms. S. with information on the empirical support of the model for treating sexual abuse–related PTSD with children, discussed the steps of treatment, and estimated that treatment might be expected to last approximately 6 months, barring any unforeseen setbacks. In addition, the clinician discussed the importance of caregiver involvement in treatment by discussing research demonstrating greater treatment response from the child when a consistent and supportive caregiver is involved. Ms. S. was initially concerned that her work schedule would interfere with her ability to regularly attend sessions. After discussing her role in providing support at home and encouraging and reinforcing Mary's use of various skills, Ms. S. decided to rearrange her work schedule and requested that her "day off" occur on the same day each week so that she could attend sessions. Weekly treatment sessions included individual sessions with Mary (30–40 minutes) and parallel sessions with Ms. S. (15–20 minutes).

TREATMENT COURSE

Psychoeducation

The first two treatment sessions focused on psychoeducation about trauma, sexual abuse, and common reactions children experience when a trauma occurs. Because Mary previously identified enjoying reading and hearing stories, the clinician decided to rely heavily on this medium throughout treatment. To begin the psychoeducation process, the clinician read Mary a storybook about a cat that experiences "a bad, sad, scary thing" and the problems he experiences afterward (*Brave Bart* [Sheppard, 1998]). In addition, the book illustrates how talking about a trauma can help improve upsetting feelings and behaviors. The clinician discussed with Mary that she had helped many other children who experienced traumatic events and that talking about the trauma over time helped them feel better. Mary appeared relieved and excited when hearing this and asked the clinician various questions, such as the age of the other children and whether they experienced feelings similar to hers. This initial portion of psychoeducation served to normalize Mary's feelings and behaviors, explain the treatment process, and instill hope that improvement was possible.

To provide psychoeducation specifically about sexual abuse, a commonly used game card was employed (*What Do You Know?* [Deblinger, Neubauer, Runyon, & Baker, 2006]). Before the session, the clinician sorted through the cards and chose those cards/questions that best fit the client's developmental level. Mary received points for attempting to answer a question (e.g., What is child sexual abuse? How do children feel when they have been sexually abused?), and extra points were awarded for the correct answer. Praise for effort was given throughout the game. The clinician discussed the answers with Mary and corrected noted misconceptions. Mary appeared relaxed and proud of her ability to answer many of these questions related to sexual abuse.

In addition, the clinician taught Mary the "safety triangle." By extending their arms downward and joining their hands together, children can create a "safety triangle" that covers the private part areas on their own body. This was used to help facilitate a discussion around private parts of the body and naming these parts of the body with the correct language. First, the clinician asked Mary to name nonsexual body parts (e.g., elbow, hand). Once Mary successfully named these parts, the clinician asked Mary whether she felt embarrassed about naming them. As expected, Mary denied feeling embarrassed. Next, the clinician discussed how all human beings have private parts with "doctor's names" and encouraged Mary to discuss the anatomical names of male and female sexual body parts. The clinician asked whether talking about these parts felt embarrassing, and Mary agreed that it was more embarrassing than the previous discussion about nonsexual body parts. Mary and the clinician discussed how many kids feel embarrassed to talk about sexual body parts, but that they are a part of all people. Mary was actively engaged throughout the psychoeducation process. She asked questions, was open to the discussions, and was excited to share what she had learned with her parents.

Ms. S. and her husband also received psychoeducation. The clinician discussed with them statistics on sexual abuse; reviewed handouts addressing common symptoms, thoughts, and feelings of children who experience sexual abuse; and provided suggestions on how they might respond to Mary's feelings and behaviors. Ms. S. reported during this time that she herself was sexually abused as a child and that she understood the common reactions and symptoms that her daughter was experiencing. She became tearful when discussing her own abuse history and blamed herself for Mary's abuse because she did not see the possible signs in her child. Ms. S. worried that Mary might be retraumatized by processing the sexual abuse she experienced. The clinician reviewed the rationale for TF-CBT, including why processing the abuse might help Mary. Ms. S. was skeptical, but agreed to continue. The clinician encouraged Ms. S. to consider receiving her own treatment to address her own past victimization.

Parenting Skills Training

Ms. S. and Mary's stepfather met with the treating clinician twice per month to address parenting skills. These sessions were separate from their daughter's counseling sessions. In addition, continued support around parenting skills were provided throughout the course of treatment, often occurring at the beginning or end of Mary's sessions.

Ms. S. and her husband reported using physical discipline methods (e.g., spanking). It was apparent that Mary's parents needed education regarding normal developmental behavior for a child of Mary's age. The clinician provided worksheets on common developmental tasks and behaviors of 7-year-old children and reviewed these with the caregivers. A primary concern was Mary's inability to regulate her anger and frustration, frequent impulsivity, and occasional bossiness. Mary's caregivers realized over time that her behaviors were common for children her age and that she was not just being "bad," as they commonly believed. In addition, the clinician explained that the prolonged sexual abuse could have negatively affected her development of emotion regulation and impulse control skills.

To address the behavioral concerns, parenting sessions initially focused on establishing a structured schedule in the home, especially at bedtime, to help Mary know what to expect and ease her transition (e.g., brushing her teeth, reading a book, arranging her stuffed animals). The clinician developed a reinforcement plan using a daily calendar to reward Mary's appropriate behaviors, including following commands and refraining from hitting and yelling; Mary and her caregivers conjointly identified appropriate reinforcers. Family rules, such as no hitting and using inside voices, as well as the consequences for breaking those rules, were clearly described for Mary.

The clinician demonstrated for the caregivers how to redirect Mary's behaviors and attention and how to implement an effective time-out sequence (see Borrego, Klinkebiel, & Gibson, Chapter 9; Baughman, Chapter 10; and Blacker, Chapter 11, this volume). The clinician also demonstrated how to use time-ins to help Mary regulate her feelings with her caregiver's assistance. A "time-in" is a technique wherein a frustrated or emotionally upset child is allowed to sit with a caregiver and express and/or regulate her emotions with the support of that caregiver.

Because Mary reported limited one-on-one time with her parents, the caregivers were encouraged to spend more time engaging with Mary in fun activities, and not use the removal of these positive interactions as consequences for problematic behavior. Ms. S. and her husband agreed to no longer use physical discipline with Mary.

Relaxation Skills Training

Two sessions focused on teaching Mary relaxation skills. First, Mary received more focused instruction on using controlled breathing exercises. The clinician taught her to identify different types of breaths through blowing different-size bubbles and helped Mary learn diaphragmatic (belly) breathing by inflating balloons at a constant speed of breath. In addition, the clinician attempted to teach Mary progressive muscle relaxation skills, but Mary found this skill uncomfortable and strange.

Mary and the clinician read a book discussing different relaxation skills, primarily guided imagery and mindfulness skills (*Peaceful Piggy Meditation* [MacLean, 2004]). Mary painted her "safe place" to use during guided imagery, choosing to paint a picture of a "bubble" that mirrored the bubbles previously used during the controlled breathing exercises. Mary was then asked to focus on her belly breathing and whether she felt comfortable enough to close her eyes. Mary agreed, and the clinician asked her to imagine a bubble floating in the air. She was asked to visualize the colors of the bubble (which she had previously painted), the changing directions that bubble took as it floated, and to imagine herself blowing the bubble in a relaxed state. Mary began to smile and her body appeared relaxed in the chair.

Mary's mother and stepfather were invited into the session so Mary could show them her "bubble" and teach them the relaxation skills she had learned. The clinician asked that Mary use these skills when feeling anxious, angry, and sad or when she experienced an intrusive memory of the sexual abuse. Mary's caregivers were asked to help Mary use these techniques throughout the day and at nighttime to help address her anxiety. Mary preferred the guided imagery technique, and it was decided that her "bubble" would be the primary coping skill used throughout upcoming therapy sessions.

Affective Identification and Modulation Training

Mary learned affect identification and modulation over the course of three sessions. Revisiting the concept of mindfulness that was previously introduced through the *Peaceful Piggy Meditation* book, music tempo was used to illustrate different mood states and physiological responses in the body. Mary was able to identify how her affect would change in response to listening to different beats, rhythms, tones, and tempos pre-chosen by the clinician. Mary was able to notice how her physical reactions would respond differently as well. Mary enjoyed this activity and afterward was able to describe how different stimuli, other than music, could impact her physiological state and affect.

Mary's understanding of the connection between physical sensations and affect was reinforced through books and art projects. First, the clinician read books with Mary to increase her vocabulary for various types of feelings (*The Way I Feel* [Cain, 2000]) and to help her understand that multiple feelings may be experienced simultaneously (*Double-Dip Feelings* [Cain, 2001]). Next, Mary participated in an activity in which she assigned a specific color to different feelings (e.g., red for anger, blue for sad). Then, using a template of a body, she colored in the body parts where she would experience different feelings within her own body. She was able to identify by name the different feelings she experienced during the sexual abuse, the feelings she experienced when remembering the sexual abuse, and the different physical locations and sensations that accompanied these feelings.

Mary was taught to use the Subjective Units of Distress (SUDs) scale to rate the intensity of her feelings. Mary practiced using the SUDs scale (0 = not at all distressing to 5 = the most intense feeling possible) with daily feelings, as well as with any feelings that emerged related to her sexual abuse. The clinician helped Mary identify which feelings, at what intensity, should prompt her to use the previously learned coping skills. To help her translate these skills to settings outside of treatment, Mary made a "coping skills envelope" that contained pictures she drew and captions that would remind her to utilize her coping skills in response to different feelings. She took this envelope home to help her manage upsetting feelings.

Multiple strategies were used to help Mary manage her distress at bedtime. First, the clinician provided psychoeducation about anxiety and how fears can be generalized to different situations. Second, Mary received a nightlight and a flashlight that she could take to bed with her, as Mary reported only seeing ghosts when it was dark. During session Mary would use the flashlight and practice turning it on to make the ghosts go away. In addition, Mary constructed a dream catcher to help her feel safe at night. Last, Mary was asked to use guided imagery at night as she went to bed and envision her "bubble" as providing a protective shield against the ghosts.

Mary taught these affect modulation skills to her caregivers and informed them of the various techniques designed to help her sleep at night. The clinician encouraged them to help Mary implement the bedtime plan each night and to help her practice her emotion identification and modulation skills at home. Mary and her caregivers often struggled to practice the skills outside of session. These issues were discussed with the clinician, and repeated attempts were made to overcome barriers by scheduling time each week to practice the skills, and developing a checklist of the different parts of the bedtime plan to be implemented each night. Despite these efforts, Mary and her caregivers continued to infrequently practice the skills at home and rarely implemented the bedtime plan.

Cognitive Coping

One session was spent teaching Mary how thoughts, feelings, and behaviors influence one another (the cognitive triangle). Initially, Mary was asked to think about an incident during the week that elicited feelings of anger, sadness, or fear. She described an incident at school in which she got into trouble for talking and became angry, which led her to yell at the teacher. The clinician asked Mary to identify her immediate thoughts when the teacher asked her to be quiet. She reported thinking that her teacher was "picking" on her and did not like her. When asked to consider alternative thoughts, Mary struggled. The clinician asked whether the teacher had ever said something similar to other children in the class, and Mary quickly agreed that she had. The clinician asked Mary whether that meant that the teacher was picking on those children and did not like them. With some discussion of this scenario, Mary came to realize that other explanations for her teacher's behavior were more appropriate, and she no longer believed that her teacher was "picking" on her.

Following this brief example, Mary was able to realize that her thoughts were affecting her feelings and behaviors. She denied feeling angry after changing her perception that her teacher was being mean to her and did not believe she would yell at the teacher if she was not angry. The cognitive triangle was reviewed using different feelings, such as fear, sadness, and anger. When the clinician was confident that Mary understood the concepts, she asked Mary to identify her thoughts, feelings, and behaviors when intrusive thoughts of the sexual abuse occurred. Mary described thinking that she was different from everyone else, causing her to feel lonely and sad. These feelings resulted in her often playing by herself and often crying. Mary was able to realize that her thought of being different was affecting how she felt and interacted with others. The clinician promised Mary that her thoughts of being different, and other thoughts related to the sexual abuse, would be addressed in upcoming sessions.

Trauma Narrative Development and Cognitive Processing

The first session of the trauma narrative phase involved reading a book describing a girl's disclosure of sexual abuse and how she overcame the impact it caused (*Please Tell! A Child's Story about Sexual Abuse* [Jessie, 1991]). When given different suggestions on how to construct her own narrative, Mary chose to write her own book "just like the girl in the story." Mary rated her SUDs score as a 4 when thinking about beginning the narrative of the abuse. However, when the clinician suggested that Mary begin by making a cover for her book and completing a simple introduction page, Mary reported her SUDs score decreased to a 1. She identified a title for her book and was able to introduce herself without notable distress. As part of the introduction Mary was asked to identify what her book would be about. She was able to verbalize that it would be an account of her sexual abuse.

During the next session Mary reviewed the work she completed previously and was asked to begin talking about her life before, during, and after the sexual abuse. Mary completed this task with minimal reported distress; however, when asked to begin discussing the sexual abuse directly, Mary's affect changed and she appeared to withdraw. She reported her SUDs score as a 5. The clinician directed Mary in the guided imagery process and encouraged her to use controlled breathing, reducing the SUDs score to a 2. The clinician refocused Mary on the narrative and asked her to complete only two sentences in relation to the sexual abuse, which Mary was able to do. The third session of the narrative construction proceeded in a similar way to the second session: Mary showed pronounced distress, but was able to develop a handful of additional sentences by using her coping skills.

During the fourth session, Mary was withdrawn. She looked down at the floor and appeared sad. When asked to resume work on her trauma narrative, Mary appeared avoidant and declined to discuss the sexual abuse any further. She reported her SUDs score as a 5. Although relaxation techniques were used in session to address Mary's distress level, she was unable to resume her trauma narrative. The clinician met with Mary's caregivers to discuss any possible changes in Mary's affect and behavior over the past week. Mary's mother suggested the change may be a result of the family maintaining contact with the aunts and uncles who were related to the perpetrator, and that these family members were unsupportive of Mary and did not believe the sexual abuse occurred. She described how those family members often treated Mary as an outcast since the disclosure, including refusing to hug and play with her as they had before. Compounding the issue was a recent decision by the district attorney to press criminal charges against the cousin. The clinician discussed concerns that the relatives' behavior might prompt Mary to experience self-blame for the stresses in the family and potentially experience regret for disclosing the sexual abuse. The clinician empathized with the difficulty that sexual abuse can cause for a family, but asserted that it was of utmost importance to keep Mary emotionally safe and not allow the family stress to prompt thoughts of self-blame or guilt. The caregivers were unwilling to completely sever contact with the nonsupportive family members, but agreed to limit contact with them and require that Mary never be left alone with them during visits.

At the next session, the clinician decided to begin relaxation techniques at the outset before the narrative was introduced owing to Mary's high SUDs score and anxiety the previous session. Mary began by blowing bubbles as a method of controlled breathing, which she enjoyed, and led her directly into use of her "bubble" guided imagery technique. Mary reported her SUDs score as a 0 after relaxation techniques were implemented. Mary and the clinician then reviewed the trauma narrative portions previously completed. Mary's SUDs score increased to a 3, but she agreed to attempt writing a few sentences and was able to successfully resume the narrative process. During the parallel session with the caregivers, Mary's mother reported that they had not visited with the unsupportive family members during the past week.

During the next four sessions, Mary engaged in relaxation techniques before proceeding with her narrative. She appeared motivated and did not report a SUDs score higher than 3. After completing the narrative, Mary and the clinician read through the account together to process her maladaptive cognitions. A recurring theme was thoughts of self-blame because she did not tell her parents sooner about the sexual abuse. Much of the delay in disclosing the abuse was a result of her believing the perpetrator was in love with her and that she was his "girlfriend," a belief promoted by the perpetrator. In addition, the cousin threatened Mary that telling others about the abuse would result in her being taken away from the family and him going to jail.

The clinician helped Mary work through these maladaptive thoughts using Socratic questioning techniques. For instance, Mary had a best friend, "Julie," and the clinician asked Mary whose fault it would be if Julie was sexually abused. Mary was also asked to consider potential feelings Julie might have about disclosing the abuse (e.g., "scared") and whether delaying a disclosure out of fear meant that Julie was at fault for the abuse. Mary was able to provide adaptive answers to these questions, at which time the clinician asked Mary to consider how her situation was different from the hypothetical situation just discussed with Julie. Mary looked puzzled for a short time, before loudly proclaiming, "It wasn't my fault at all."

The clinician shared the newly developed portions of the trauma narrative with Mary's caregivers during each session. Hearing portions of the trauma narrative were noticeably difficult for Ms. S., but she was able to discuss her thoughts on Mary's sexual abuse, including her own self-blame for failing to recognize the "signs" of sexual abuse. The clinician used Socratic questioning methods similar to those used with Mary to address Ms. S.'s thoughts of self-blame. An example of a puzzle, without an accompanying picture, was used as an analogy for Ms. S. not seeing the "signs" of sexual abuse. The clinician described that isolated behaviors (i.e., "pieces of the puzzle") may be present, but without knowing the context in which those behaviors occurred (i.e., "knowledge of the complete picture"), it becomes incredibly difficult to correctly understand the connection, or "put the pieces together."

Ms. S. was able to change her thoughts of self-blame into thoughts of regret that her daughter had experienced sexual abuse. The clinician empathized with Ms. S. that Mary's experience was unfortunate, but stressed that it is more helpful to concentrate on the present and future rather than focusing on the past. Ms. S. agreed and noted how Mary's emotional and behavioral concerns were significantly improved since beginning treatment.

The caregivers believed they were ready to hear the narrative from Mary herself, and the clinician discussed with them the process of Mary sharing the trauma narrative. The clinician emphasized the importance of Ms. S. remaining composed during the conjoint session, as significant distress from her could result in Mary becoming sad and feeling guilty for upsetting her mother. The clinician encouraged Ms. S. and Mary's stepfather to use active listening and state how proud they were of Mary for telling her story. The caregivers denied having any specific questions they wanted to ask Mary during the conjoint session. Ms. S. added that Mary still had not seen the unsupportive aunts and uncles.

In Vivo Exposure

Mary previously reported that she would become anxious and think about the sexual abuse when seeing red SUVs. The clinician provided education on how trauma reminders can trigger fearful reactions and how guided imagery and controlled breathing can be used to address this trauma reminder. First, Mary was asked to imagine any type of car in any color. This exercise did not cause her anxiety. Next, she was asked to imagine only red cars, at which time Mary's SUDs level increased to 3. At this point the clinician asked Mary to focus on her controlled breathing. Mary did so and reported a significant reduction in anxiety. The clinician then prompted Mary to again imagine a red car, but the anxiety did not increase as before. During the next session Mary was asked to repeat the above procedure and this time reported no SUDs scores higher than 1. Noting this improvement, the clinician then instructed Mary to think of a red SUV. Mary reported her SUDs level at 4 and self-initiated controlled breathing techniques, which reduced her SUDs level to 2. Mary was asked to work on using her controlled breathing and guided imagery when seeing a red car, an SUV, or a red SUV outside of session. Within two sessions, Mary reported no longer being afraid of red SUVs and was so proud that she had her mother take a picture of her standing next to one in a parking lot. No *in vivo* experiences occurred with the polka-dot patterned skirt, as the family had given it away because it was now too small for Mary.

Conjoint Caregiver–Child Session

Mary did not appear nervous or avoidant when sharing her narrative with her caregivers. Mary's mother actively listened during the recitation of the narrative and provided encouraging comments throughout. At one point Ms. S. became slightly tearful, but was able to remain supportive and composed. At the conclusion of Mary reading her narrative, Ms. S. stated how proud she was of Mary for completing her narrative and agreed that the abuse was not her fault. During the following session, Mary told the clinician how proud she was of herself and that she felt supported by her mother and stepfather. Ms. S. reported that she and her husband decided to permanently sever ties with the unsupportive family members because of their continued lack of support for Mary and the manner in which they treated her.

Enhance Safety and Future Development

The last few sessions focused on teaching Mary safety skills and preparing her for treatment termination. The clinician and Mary read a book about a pigeon that attempts to coerce the reader to do various things by pleading, becoming angry and making threats, and offering rewards (*Don't Let the Pigeon Drive the Bus* [Willems, 2003]). The clinician used the story to teach Mary ways to say "No" when dealing with general life events, especially if someone asks Mary to engage in sexual behaviors. Using role-play exercises, Mary actively practiced using these assertiveness skills.

Mary completed a safety plan worksheet with the treating clinician. This worksheet identified what Mary would do if someone tried to sexually abuse her or made her feel uncomfortable, whom she could tell, what to do if that person did not believe her, and ways to keep herself safe. Mary and the clinician reviewed these safety skills with Ms. S., and Mary explained the safety plan to her mother. The clinician made a copy of the completed worksheet for Mary to take home.

Mary reported feeling much better than when she began treatment, but was sad about the prospect of not seeing the clinician anymore. The clinician read Mary a book addressing feelings about discharging from treatment (*The Invisible String* [Karst, 2000]). The book illustrates how people are still bonded with other people even though they may not see each other anymore. Mary and the clinician both made a bracelet out of yarn and exchanged bracelets with each other to represent the invisible string that binds them.

TREATMENT COMPLETION

Treatment comprised 23 sessions. Both Mary and her caregivers reported a significant decrease in her symptoms and believed that she was doing well overall. Mary no longer complained of seeing ghosts or having frequent nightmares, and described feeling happy and closer to her family. Ms. S. completed another UCLA PTSD Reaction Index, and noticeable improvements were observed. It was decided at this time that treatment was complete. During the final session Mary decided to write a letter to other children to encourage them to complete their trauma narrative.

COMMENTARY

At first glance, this case appears to be a reasonably standard example of child sexual abuse, if there is such a thing. The child had a minimal trauma history other than sexual abuse by an adult relative and displayed symptoms and problems that are common among CSA victims, including reexperiencing, avoidance, hyperarousal, fears, anxiety, depression, and moderate behavior problems. It was an ideal case for TF-CBT, and results of TF-CBT outcome studies suggest her prognosis was good to excellent. However, the case illustrates several clinical choice points, timing and pacing issues, and technique choices that often occur in a course of TF-CBT, even with a relatively straightforward case. These are discussed below.

Perceived Safety

This young girl demonstrated problems with her perceived sense of safety. She was generally withdrawn and somewhat anxious, had an exaggerated startle response, and was hypervigilant, all signs of fear activation and safety concerns. The therapist verbally reassured Mary that she was safe in the therapy room, but her fear and anxiety were elevated to the point that the therapist taught her controlled breathing skills in order to continue the initial session. This situation of high fear and anxiety raises an important clinical question for a therapist using TF-CBT: when should extensive safety planning be incorporated into the very early sessions of treatment rather than at the end as described in the TF-CBT PRACTICE component model?

In a recent report on a clinical trial using TF-CBT with children exposed to intimate partner violence, many of whom were still living in the violent home, Cohen and colleagues (Cohen, Mannarino, & Iyengar, 2011) suggested that in cases wherein real threats to a child's safety continue to exist during treatment, safety planning should be the initial component of TF-CBT. The decision to make this change in the standard protocol depends on the nature and seriousness of genuine threats to safety, which would be revealed by a detailed safety assessment.

One could argue that a child's perceived sense of danger should trigger such a change in protocol as well. At the least, a thorough safety assessment should be conducted to better understand the source of the child's above-average fears. In some cases, the fears actually may be the result of an accurate assessment of a situation by the child rather than misperceptions, inaccurate interpretations of situations, or maladaptive thinking that may be targets of therapy.

In Mary's case, the therapist learned in the course of treatment that the family was continuing to have contact with close family members of the offender who did not believe the abuse occurred and were angry at the child for making the allegations. The child rightly viewed this situation as dangerous and was reacting to it. Upon learning of the circumstances, the therapist appropriately intervened and worked with the family to develop a safety plan to reduce the child's contact with these family members. Ideally, such a situation is detected during the assessment phase. In cases of abuse wherein the offender is a relative, it is common for other family members to not believe the child, be convinced the offender is innocent, and be angry at the child. Asking about such situations should be included as part of a safety assessment. After learning of the relatives' anger, a safety plan can be put in place at that point and potentially reduce the likelihood of interrupting treatment at a later time.

Parental Engagement and Involvement

Parental involvement in treatment is a key element of TF-CBT and virtually all evidence-based treatments for children. Consequently, it is crucial that effective engagement strategies be used to gain the parent's support and participation. As part of the engagement process with Mary's caregivers, the therapist gave the parents information about TF-CBT, emphasized how important it was that they participate, and worked with them to problem-solve several obstacles they brought up, including work schedules. Through these efforts, the clinician was able to achieve regular parental involvement in session. An effective tactic the therapist used in this case was to emphasize the time-limited nature of TF-CBT. Many parents of sexually abused children worry that their child may need treatment for a very long time, even "the rest of her life." Explaining that TF-CBT usually is completed in a few months (8–24 weeks) is normally a surprise to them. Whatever adjustments need to be made in work, school, or other schedules will be relatively short term and therefore more feasible.

The case description indicated that the child's mother rearranged her work schedule so she could consistently bring the child to therapy on her day off. Even given the relatively short duration of TF-CBT, many parents do not have the luxury of a regular day off during the work week, and taking a full day off work to bring a child to a weekly 60- to 90-minute therapy session is not practical for most people. Parents (and employers) often agree to rearrange work schedules to get the child to therapy at the time of the initial crisis of disclosure. However, after a few weeks, and after the crisis subsides, these arrangements can become burdensome and result in more sporadic attendance. Therapists should work with parents to develop practical arrangements for therapy that can be sustained over the full course of treatment. For example, could parents take a half day or a few hours off of work each week, if needed? Could late afternoon or evening appointments be arranged to reduce work and school conflicts?

In several of the parent sessions, it was reported that the child taught the newly learned skills to the parents. It is important to emphasize that Mary "taught" the skills to her parents, rather than simply demonstrated them. Teaching has several benefits over demonstrations. First, the child gains a sense of empowerment and better mastery of the skills through this process. Second, parents learn how to participate in a child-directed (vs. parent-directed) interaction with their child. This parenting skill is difficult for many parents. Finally, parents are more likely to learn the skill if they have to do it in session, which better sets up the family for practice at home.

Also in the case report, the parents were described as rarely helping Mary practice the skills at home or implementing the bedtime plan to help with sleep problems. Lack of parental cooperation with home practice or new routines is a frequent problem in treatment. Mary's therapist tried many approaches to gaining parental cooperation with little success, which can be frustrating and reduce the positive effects of treatment. Another approach that might encourage parental cooperation is to essentially put the parents on a token economy for their practice behavior, much like they do with their child. Therapists might consider using behavior charts, tokens, and rewards with parents to encourage their cooperation at home. This technique has the added benefit of teaching the parents how to properly set up and execute a token economy with their child. Another method is to use between-session phone calls, e-mail, or text messages to remind parents to practice with their child. Some phone and e-mail systems can be programmed to do this automatically at specifically agreed-upon times. When reminders such as these are used, it removes the "I forgot" excuse, and the therapist can focus fully on the parent's choice to simply not do the practice assignments.

Gradual Exposure during PRAC Components

This case report indicates that the therapist did a good job teaching the PRAC skills in a creative and effective manner; however, it appears that the application of these skills to Mary's memories of her own sexual abuse were not a specific focus of the PRAC components. The clinician did discuss Mary's own abuse in numerous places, such as encouraging her to use the relaxation skills when she remembers the abuse or identifying her thoughts and feelings related to the abuse, but high levels of distress and resistance associated with beginning the trauma narrative may suggest that gradual exposure was not incorporated to a sufficient degree during the PRAC components. Remembering that gradual exposure to one's trauma should be an integral part of each component of TF-CBT, the trauma narrative should be a natural extension of the therapy, rather than a sudden shock. Mary's difficulty engaging in the trauma narrative appears to have been due, at least partially, to her ongoing fear related to her disbelieving family members. However, increased use of gradual exposure during the PRAC phases of treatment may have improved her ability to more efficiently develop the trauma narrative.

In Vivo Exposure

Mary had several specific trauma triggers (e.g., red SUVs, polka-dot skirt) that could be managed using *in vivo* exposure. The therapist chose to initially use covert desensitization, rather than true *in vivo* exposure, by having the child imagine the trauma triggers and use relaxation and other calming skills to reduce anxiety. This approach seems to have worked for this child, as it laid the foundation for her being able to directly confront the previously feared red SUVs in the physical world. *In vivo* exposure is the real-life, direct confrontation of feared objects, activities, or situations, rather than imaginal exposure conducted in the therapy room (Rothbaum et al., 2006). Both can be effective. There can be times when true *in vivo* exposure is necessary to gain the real-life reduction in anxiety, so the TF-CBT therapist should be prepared to use it when necessary.

Summary

Although this case initially appeared to be a straightforward case of TF-CBT, it illustrates several common challenges that TF-CBT therapists may need to manage. First, TF-CBT therapists should be prepared to conduct a thorough safety assessment when children present with greater than average fears and be prepared to conduct safety planning when necessary at any point during treatment. Effectively engaging parents in the treatment and ensuring sufficient gradual exposure throughout the early components of treatment are key elements of TF-CBT. Last, while imaginal exposure can be effective, *in vivo* exposure should be used when necessary.

REFERENCES

Cain, B. (2001). *Double-dip feelings*. Washington, DC: Magination Press.

Cain, J. (2000). *The way I feel*. Seattle, WA: Parenting Press.

Cohen, J. A., Mannarino, A. P., & Iyengar, S. (2011). Community treatment of posttraumatic stress disorder for children exposed to intimate partner violence: A randomized controlled trial. *Archives of Pediatrics and Adolescent Medicine, 165*(1), 16–21.

Deblinger, E., Neubauer, F., Runyon, M., & Baker, D. (2006). *What do you know?: A therapeutic card game about child sexual and physical abuse and domestic violence*. Stratford, NJ: CARES Institute, University of Medicine and Dentistry of New Jersey.

Jessie. (1991). *Please tell!: A child's story about sexual abuse*. Center City, MN: Hazelden.

Karst, P. (2000). *The invisible string*. Camarillo, CA: DeVorss.

MacLean, K. L. (2004). *Peaceful piggy meditation*. Chicago: Whitman.

Rothbaum, B. O., Anderson, P., Zimand, E., Hodges, L., Lang, D., & Wilson, J. (2006). Virtual reality exposure therapy and standard (in vivo) exposure therapy in the treatment of fear of flying. *Behavior Therapy, 37*(1), 80–90.

Sheppard, C. H. (1998). *Brave Bart: A story for traumatized and grieving children*. Grosse Point Woods, MI: Institute for Trauma and Loss in Children.

Steinberg, A. M., Brymer, M. J., Decker, K. B., & Pynoos, R. S. (2004). The University of California at Los Angeles PTSD Reaction Index. *Current Psychiatry Reports, 6*, 96–100.

Willems, M. (2003). *Don't let the pigeon drive the bus!* New York: Hyperion.

5

TF-CBT with a School-Age Boy with a History of Neglect and Witnessing Domestic Violence

The Case of Gabriel S.

Alexandra Tellez

with commentary by Benjamin E. Saunders

BACKGROUND INFORMATION

Gabriel S. is a Hispanic boy who was 9 years old when he presented for treatment at a community-based outpatient clinic. He was referred by Ms. R., an older cousin with whom he lived, following unsuccessful treatment with another clinician. At the time of the intake assessment, Gabriel was reported to display irritability, occasional aggression toward others, seeming to always be on "alert mode," and was very sensitive to noises around him, such as loudly shutting doors or occasional loud play by his younger siblings. Gabriel experienced uncontrollable anger outbursts demonstrated by his need to punch pillows, throw himself against the wall, and throw objects. Of greatest concern to the family was Gabriel's tendency to bang his head against the wall or cement floors during periods of frustration and anger. He usually was unwilling to take responsibility for his misbehavior, would steal or hide family possessions, and was cruel to animals. Previous services primarily utilized nondirective play therapy and occurred over the course of 1 year.

ASSESSMENT AND TREATMENT PLANNING

Gabriel's first years of life involved living in a tumultuous household where he experienced neglect by his biological mother, observed physical abuse toward a younger sibling, was exposed to pornography, and witnessed escalating domestic violence between his biological parents, partially as a result of significant substance abuse. At the age of 5, child protective services (CPS) placed Gabriel and his siblings under the care of his grandparents and Ms. R. Gabriel maintained occasional supervised visitation with his biological father, but his mother was living in a residential drug abuse treatment facility and he was unable to have contact with her.

Gabriel presented as a timid and guarded 9-year-old boy who initially struggled with disclosing information about his past. He was much more willing to talk about his younger siblings and how he continued to care for them. With respect to his parents, Gabriel expressed mixed emotions as he described missing them, but also wished that they were not violent toward each other and hoped he would have the power to stop them from hurting each other. When directly asked about the traumatic events he experienced, Gabriel would change the topic, his face would immediately flush, and he would avoid making eye contact by looking at the floor. Due to Gabriel's resistance in talking about his past, Ms. R. provided much of the information during the assessment.

Caregiver rating scales were administered to supplement the information gathered during the assessment interview. Ms. R. completed the Behavior Assessment System for Children, Second Edition (BASC-2; Reynolds & Kamphaus, 2004), as well as the Trauma Symptom Checklist for Young Children (TSCYC; Briere, 2005). Results across both instruments were consistent in identifying elevated levels of anxiety, depression, and anger, which were expected given the reported concerns of emotional dysregulation and aggression. In addition, TSCYC posttraumatic stress avoidance and arousal scales were elevated ($T = 74$ and 75, respectively), which was consistent with Gabriel's reluctance to discuss his traumatic experiences. Gabriel was diagnosed with posttraumatic stress disorder (PTSD).

Trauma-focused cognitive-behavioral therapy (TF-CBT) was chosen as the treatment approach, as it possesses significant empirical support for treating children experiencing posttraumatic stress and other emotional and behavioral problems resulting from traumatic events. The treating clinician was a doctoral student in a clinical psychology program under the supervision and instruction of a clinical psychologist with substantial training and experience using TF-CBT. Treatment occurred once per week with individual sessions with Gabriel (30–40 minutes) and parallel sessions (10–20 minutes) with Ms. R. Including Ms. R. in session appeared the most appropriate approach for Gabriel, as his grandmother displayed significant resistance toward therapy and was unwilling to implement the interventions. His grandmother's resistance appeared attributable to cultural and religious beliefs, as she viewed mental illness as a character weakness and believed spirituality and prayer were enough to strengthen them and relieve any physical or psychological affliction. However Ms. R., while holding similar cultural and religious views, believed Gabriel needed "professional" services in addition to prayer. She was apologetic for the grandmother's refusal to participate in treatment and expressed a desire for the grandmother to be more "open minded." A significant motivation for Ms. R. was her own history of childhood trauma and a fear that Gabriel would grow up with many of the challenges she faced herself.

TREATMENT COURSE

Psychoeducation

The first three sessions of treatment focused on providing psychoeducation to normalize Gabriel's reactions to the traumatic events he experienced. The diagnosis of PTSD was explained to Gabriel's grandmother and Ms. R. Handouts in their native language (Spanish) were used to provide a general definition of the disorder and to help identify symptoms that were relevant in Gabriel's case (e.g., anger outbursts and hypervigilance). The handouts served to illustrate that other children like Gabriel experience similar symptoms.

To help Gabriel understand his symptoms, he and the clinician collaboratively read a psychoeducational storybook about a raccoon that experiences a traumatic event (*A Terrible Thing Happened* [Holmes, 2000]). Gabriel acknowledged experiencing many of the symptoms mentioned in the story, such as feelings of anger, regretting aggressive outbursts, sadness, and headaches. Although the specific trauma experienced by the raccoon is never identified in the storybook, the clinician asked Gabriel to discuss his own traumatic experiences and consider that the symptoms he endorsed were similarly related to traumatic events he experienced. Although still reluctant, Gabriel was able to provide more details of his own trauma history. A rationale for TF-CBT was provided to Gabriel, who learned that therapy involved talking about his emotions, including negative feelings about his past, and learning coping skills to deal with his reactions. He cautiously agreed to participate.

Parenting Skills Training

As a result of scheduling conflicts, Ms. R. was only able to bring Gabriel to treatment every other week, with Gabriel's grandmother accompanying him the other weeks. Despite efforts to engage the grandmother in the treatment process, she continued to refuse to participate. Therefore, the clinician met with Ms. R. on a biweekly basis to discuss Gabriel's progress in therapy, to inform her of the coping skills he was expected to practice at home and in school, and to assist her in coping with her own personal reactions to Gabriel's disclosure of past traumatic experiences. Ms. R. often became tearful as she recalled the violent encounters between Gabriel's biological parents and the level of neglect to which he was exposed. Session time was dedicated to help her process her reactions, such as the anger and resentment she "bottled up" against Gabriel's parents. She was encouraged to seek her own psychological services to better cope with the daily stressors of caring for Gabriel and improve her life and work balance, as she held a demanding job.

The meetings with Ms. R. also were used to teach her specific child behavior management skills to help deal with Gabriel's stealing, lying, and aggressive play with other children. More specifically, it became necessary to explain to Ms. R. how important it was to praise Gabriel for positive behaviors or potential signs of improvement, no matter how small the change (e.g., completing a chore without being asked to or his immediate response to commands). As she started to implement these skills, Ms. R. realized that she was spending more time praising Gabriel for his positive changes than reprimanding him for his problematic behavior. The clinician encouraged her to "choose her battles" and to categorize Gabriel's behavior into the activities that absolutely could not be ignored (e.g., stealing), and the emotions she could live with or "let pass" for the day (e.g. Gabriel's occasional irritability). In addition, the clinician helped Ms. R. understand the importance of remaining consistent with the consequences she outlined for Gabriel's stealing, lying and aggressive behaviors toward others.

A behavioral intervention that was particularly effective with Gabriel was the use of a visible behavior chart that tracked his weekly progress in meeting behavioral goals. This chart was taped to the refrigerator door and Ms. R. implemented a points reward system in which Gabriel would "cash out" his points on a weekly basis for small treats (e.g., ice cream, extra time playing outside). Other recommendations included increased monitoring of Gabriel and decreasing opportunities for him to engage in problematic behaviors, such as securing valuable items to prevent stealing.

Gabriel described himself as deeply religious and enjoyed reading the Bible. Given his interests in biblical scriptures, the clinician recommended that Ms. R. use Bible verses to help him consider and understand his wrongdoings. In addition, Gabriel enjoyed teaching others about biblical passages, and allowing him to read verses during the family's weekly religious meetings served as a way to reward the positive strides in his behavior.

Relaxation Skills Training

Four sessions were dedicated to teaching Gabriel relaxation skills. A balloon of his choosing was used to illustrate the concept of controlled breathing. As he took deep breaths of air, he was asked to imagine he had the small balloon inside his belly slowly inflating. Similarly, when he exhaled through the mouth he was asked to imagine a balloon slowly deflating. A quickly deflating balloon was used to demonstrate what happens when a person loses control of his or her breathing. For example, as the air went all over the place, a person's uncontrolled breathing may also make him or her feel out of control. Gabriel was easily engaged in this activity, and he became excited when asked to demonstrate his mastery of the "cool air" technique. A second activity required him to fully recline in his chair and place a cup on his lower abdomen to see it go up and down (referred to as "belly breathing" for Gabriel). This technique was used to gauge Gabriel's ability to breathe using his diaphragm.

Progressive muscle relaxation techniques were demonstrated by providing concrete examples for each muscle group. For instance, Gabriel was asked to imagine he was squeezing and letting go of a lemon to practice relaxing forearm and hand muscles and being a turtle in a shell where he would pull his head into his shoulders and then out again thereby tensing and relaxing his shoulder muscles. In addition, Gabriel completed a positive imagery exercise, which he referred to as the "happy place." Gabriel's "happy place" was going to the beach with his siblings. Gabriel drew a picture of him and his siblings at the beach and provided details describing the weather, the topics of play and conversation, and his feelings, as well as the feelings of his siblings. Gabriel displayed a large smile throughout this activity, and the clinician pointed out that recounting the beach story appeared to make him happy. Gabriel agreed.

The clinician instructed Gabriel to practice all of these skills and envision them as elements in his "toolbox." He was to rely on them when he felt angry or sad, when he thought about his prior traumatic experiences, and even when he could not quite explain what he was feeling. Although Gabriel took pride in these skills, he initially failed to practice them at home. He expressed concern that others would judge him as doing them incorrectly. His fear to practice them in front of others decreased when he was reminded that it would be difficult for others to judge him if they were not trained in the techniques and did not have access to his toolbox. He taught each of these skills to Ms. R., who praised Gabriel's accomplishments and agreed to practice the skills with him at home.

Another challenge was for Gabriel to remember that he could utilize these relaxation skills during school. Ms. R. and the clinician devised reminders to use the skills, such as a picture of a balloon, which Gabriel was able to tape to the surface of his desk. The clinician and Ms. R. consistently praised Gabriel for his positive behavioral reports from school and his own statements that he was utilizing the skills. With time and practice, Gabriel became more efficient at mastering the skills across multiple settings.

Affective Identification and Modulation Training

Two sessions were devoted to teaching Gabriel affective identification and modulation skills. First, to expand his emotional vocabulary, Gabriel and the clinician reviewed a feelings poster that described various feelings that one may experience. He was surprised to learn individuals can sometimes experience more than one feeling at the same time. His mixed feelings toward his biological parents were used as an example, as he explained both loving and being angry with them. This was followed by playing a game that involved labeling photographs of faces expressing different feelings. He enjoyed the game and was encouraged to review the feelings poster for clues to the answers.

Second, Gabriel was taught to rate the intensity of emotions using a subjective units of distress (SUDs) scale, ranging from 1 (low intensity) to 10 (most intense feeling). Gabriel and the clinician discussed the scale as a sort of thermometer to help him determine when he should use his coping skills toolbox to improve his mood. To provide concrete experiences in the use of the SUDs scale and emotion identification skills, the clinician asked Gabriel to consider the type and intensity of his feelings when he thinks about his parents and his experiences of neglect and witnessing violence. Gabriel stated that he usually is angry and rated the anger as a "9 or 10." The clinician then prompted Gabriel to use skills from his toolbox to reduce the intensity of his anger.

Given Gabriel's treatment history with nondirective play therapy, he was often excited to participate in games and play activities as various TF-CBT techniques were introduced. These approaches, such as emotional bingo, role playing, and guessing the severity of emotions portrayed, were used to teach and reinforce concepts. For example, the latter activity involved the clinician and Gabriel making faces and taking turns (1) guessing the emotion and (2) providing a SUDs rating representing the intensity of the emotion displayed. Gabriel was able to improve his ability to identify and verbalize how he felt in different situations as well as use relaxation skills when he identified feeling angry, frustrated, or misunderstood.

At this point in treatment Gabriel began to show signs that he was wavering in his motivation to participate. He would make comparisons between his treating clinician and his previous play therapist, suggesting that this new therapy involved "too much work and not enough playing time." Although he believed that the treatment was helping, he missed the unstructured play that he previously enjoyed. The clinician provided additional psychoeducation regarding why TF-CBT required active participation on his part, but added that his participation would now be rewarded with unstructured play time during the last 10 minutes of each session. Gabriel was skilled at crafts, and his unstructured play time primarily involved working on various art projects, mostly pieces he would make for his siblings, grandparents, and Ms. R.

Cognitive Coping

While transitioning into the cognitive coping phase, Gabriel started acting out at school by arguing and instigating fights with his peers. These setbacks in his behavior were likely precipitated by the instability he was experiencing at home. Due to financial stressors, Gabriel's grandparents lost their home and moved in with Ms. R. Gabriel no longer had privacy, as he was now sleeping in the same room with his siblings and Ms. R.'s 12-year-old son. Time was spent emphasizing how he could use his relaxation skills to cope during particularly stressful times, even those that were not related to negative feelings about his past.

Gabriel was involved in a physical altercation with a peer at school, resulting in a 2-day in-school suspension. This event was used in session to illustrate the concept of cognitive coping. Gabriel had difficulty discussing his thoughts, and initially was only able to discuss his feelings and behaviors surrounding this event. When asked what he was thinking when the boy bumped into him and his friend, Gabriel responded by discussing alternate behaviors or different ways he could have reacted. He also said that he could have told a teacher the boy was bothering him, or he could have just ignored him and walked away. He was able to identify the anger and embarrassment he was feeling at the moment. Gabriel expressed how challenging it was for him to not feel angry and struggled to verbalize what was maintaining that anger. After going over the event a third time and drawing an illustration, Gabriel realized that he was not only angry, but also believed he was acting in self-defense to protect a close friend.

Given that Gabriel struggled to differentiate between his thoughts and feelings, time was spent clarifying the two by using a handout that required him to match various thoughts to corresponding feelings. One column of this handout listed various feelings, such as guilty, hopeful, angry, and happy. The second column had thought phrases that were related to each feeling (e.g., "my friends like me," which was to be matched with "happy"). After this handout was completed, the cognitive triangle was introduced by having him illustrate the altercation and the other children involved. A thought bubble (i.e., a large circle) was drawn next to each boy's face for Gabriel to write some possible thoughts that he and his friend had and possible alternative thoughts. Gabriel then considered how these different thoughts would have led to different feelings and subsequent behaviors. Once Gabriel demonstrated mastery of the cognitive coping skills, the clinician discussed that the same techniques would be used to process unhelpful thoughts he may have about his prior traumatic experiences.

Trauma Narrative Development and Cognitive Processing

As is often the case, writing the trauma narrative proved to be the most challenging part of treatment for Gabriel. The construction of his narrative took several weeks, as he began refusing to attend treatment because of how difficult he anticipated it would be to discuss his past. He resisted by throwing tantrums when it was time to leave his home for sessions and expressed anger about the prospect of talking about his mother. Initially, Gabriel was persuaded to come to treatment by Ms. R.'s promise of taking him to his favorite fast-food restaurant after the session. During these first sessions of the trauma narrative, the clinician reviewed the psychoeducational storybook about the raccoon and how talking about his past experiences resulted in the raccoon's improvement. The clinician also reviewed the coping skills (e.g., relaxation training and positive imagery) learned and the importance of Gabriel identifying when to pause and use his toolbox to cope with upsetting feelings. Although it was important for Gabriel to understand he was leading the construction of the narrative, the clinician also reserved the right to pause when Gabriel demonstrated any signs of distress (e.g., flushed face and teary eyes). Gabriel was more at ease after discussing these issues, and Ms. R.'s fast food incentive was only required for 2 weeks.

Before much progress was made on the construction of the narrative, several sessions were missed because of issues at home that required CPS involvement. Gabriel and his siblings were removed from his maternal grandparents and Ms. R. and temporarily assigned to the care of another relative following an allegation of sexual abuse by one of his siblings against an uncle. Two weeks later, due to financial reasons, the children were separated and only Gabriel was relocated to a new foster home. It took a few weeks for Gabriel to adjust to this new home and resume treatment sessions. Fortunately, Gabriel had excelled in expanding his feelings vocabulary, and he identified feelings of guilt and loneliness as he struggled over the separation from his siblings. During his earlier experiences of neglect, he often assumed the responsibility of feeding himself and his siblings by opening cans of food without his parents' permission. Not surprisingly, he expressed worry over not having dinner with his siblings, as he feared they would not have enough to eat. Talking to them on the phone before bed and knowing they were safe and happy relieved these concerns.

Two sessions were dedicated to helping Gabriel cope with adjusting to the new foster home and the other children in the house. Gabriel's foster parents were very supportive of him attending treatment and requested to change the weekly sessions to another day in the week that would accommodate both Ms. R. and the foster mother's work schedule. Despite the change in living arrangement, Gabriel did not regress to his previous patterns of misbehavior and formed a supportive and trusting relationship with the foster mother. However, Gabriel's foster parents often compared him to their own children, which initially made it difficult for them to comprehend why Gabriel displayed occasional irritability and frustration. The clinician discussed with the foster parents basic principles of child development and the impact child maltreatment can exert on coping and interpersonal skills. The foster parents displayed greater empathy and understanding toward Gabriel, and the clinician recommended that the foster parents continue using the behavioral chart, which had proven effective in his previous home. Overall, Gabriel was generally excited to have his own room, not have to share a bed, and have his own "space to play." Although he was able to see his siblings at school, he nonetheless missed them very much and reported thinking of his "happy place," playing with his siblings on the beach, on a daily basis.

After these few sessions to help with the transition to a foster home, the construction of the trauma narrative continued. The narrative was a very intimidating task for Gabriel, especially because his first response when discussing his past with his biological parents was to avoid talking about it, either by changing the subject or remaining silent. Gabriel had mentioned numerous times previously that he wished he could change what happened to him and his siblings. To place him more at ease and allow him to exert some sense of control over the narrative, he was allowed to choose the order in which the traumatic events would be discussed and processed.

Gabriel elected to start the narrative with what he perceived as the least-threatening event, an occasion when he and a sibling witnessed their father watching pornography. Around this time, Gabriel no longer appeared dismissive of conversations about his feelings and thoughts surrounding the events. It is possible he was less avoidant in discussing his past because he was often reminded he had the power to "wave the magic wand" when he felt uncomfortable and pause to use his coping toolbox. Each session involved having Gabriel review the narrative he constructed in the previous weeks, and noticeably less avoidance was observed during each review of the previously constructed portions.

In constructing the narrative, Gabriel chose to provide a verbal account of the events while the clinician wrote down his version. Once Gabriel finished dictating a page in the narrative, he would draw a scene graphically depicting what he recounted. Gabriel referred to the drawing as the "fun part," although he quickly realized the drawing was not as fun as he expected. He did well with the illustrations, but found it difficult to draw his biological parents. Given that Gabriel was open to sharing details of their appearance, the clinician asked whether she might draw them. Gabriel agreed, and the clinician did a purposefully poor job to motivate him to help with the drawing. In fact, Gabriel disliked one of the images so much that he decided to start over and draw the complete image himself.

As Gabriel continued discussing particularly painful events, he became apologetic over not finding the most appropriate words and not having enough to say. The clinician encouraged him and thanked him for his cooperation and for the effort he was investing in the narrative. Gabriel was asked whether he would prefer for the clinician to provide detailed questions to help him along with the narrations. For example, at one point the clinician asked, "What was going through your mind when you saw your dad grab the glass vase?" Gabriel responded positively to this suggestion and eventually found enough words that he needed little guidance to discuss what he was thinking or feeling during the events.

While constructing his narrative, Gabriel was very descriptive of his environment, but he would often take long pauses before discussing his biological parents. During the long pauses he was asked to identify his feelings and to share his number on the SUDs scale. The first time this occurred, Gabriel described his feeling as angry and labeled the intensity as an 8. The clinician asked whether he thought it might be a good idea to take out his toolbox. He declined to use any of the relaxation skills and wanted to rush through his descriptions and "get this over with." The clinician discussed that the goal was to desensitize Gabriel to his traumatic memories, not rush through as quickly as possible. Gabriel agreed to use his "happy place" technique to improve his tolerance of the memories, and he said his number was now a 6. The clinician praised Gabriel for his efforts. This process was repeated numerous times during the writing of his narrative.

Gabriel displayed the most distress while recounting the domestic violence he witnessed. He described feeling helpless and guilty for not doing anything to stop his parents from hurting each other. The clinician encouraged him to focus on expressing his reasons for feeling guilty, which he identified as self-blame for not diverting or interrupting his parents. The clinician asked Gabriel to consider the possible outcomes of his getting involved in his parents' altercations. He was able to quickly reply that he may have been severely injured, just as his mother had been numerous times. He replied, "I guess that would have been worse because no one else would have cared for my siblings." Furthermore, he stated that he would have felt horrible if he had left his siblings as a result of being injured. The clinician expressed her admiration for the bravery and strength he displayed in caring for his siblings during those difficult times. With further processing, Gabriel was able to state that his involvement most likely would not have ended the domestic violence. When it was finished, Gabriel's narrative included watching pornography with a younger sibling, witnessing his mother abuse substances, sneaking into the kitchen at night to steal food from the pantry, seeing his parents engage in domestic violence toward each other, and the physical abuse of a younger sibling.

The last portion of each session was devoted to having the clinician share with Ms. R. the newly constructed sections of the narrative. This was especially important for Ms. R. given how emotionally upsetting Gabriel's past was for her personally, and to ensure she could tolerate any comments or questions Gabriel may have brought up during the conjoint session. She was amazed at the level of detail Gabriel provided for all of the events. She had assumed that Gabriel did not remember many of the events as he rarely mentioned them at home. The clinician reviewed with her that avoidance is a typical PTSD symptom, and that there was a difference between avoidance and forgetting. Ms. R. was reminded of the importance of supporting Gabriel as he shared his narrative with her during the upcoming conjoint session.

In Vivo Exposure

Gabriel was removed from the care of both of his biological parents and maintained occasional contact only with his father. Despite his maltreatment history, he described a positive relationship with his father and hoped to be reunited with him. Although his father was the primary aggressor in the domestic violence incidents, which Gabriel identified as the most distressing events for him, Gabriel maintained love and respect for him. These feelings were conflicted, however, because he also expressed disappointment toward him, while hoping he could one day share the narrative during a visit with his father. Gabriel was observed to be in a bad mood during the weeks his father made contact with him (mostly by speaking with him over the telephone), and identified feeling guilty about the anger he held toward his father.

Two approaches were used to help Gabriel cope with his distress and conflicted feelings. First, he was reminded he had unlimited access to his coping toolbox every time he encountered someone or something that reminded him of his past experiences. A list of trauma reminders, including phone discussions with his father, was constructed, and the clinician helped Gabriel develop a coping plan for each reminder on the list. Gabriel was able to identify the most appropriate coping skills from his toolbox to implement for each reminder.

Second, the concept of mixed feelings was reinforced. Explaining mixed feelings was important as Gabriel once mentioned to Ms. R. that he had a strong aversion toward his mother. He would become visibly angry in response to reminders of his mother (e.g., seeing a picture of her or hearing her name), a reaction that created further distress for him because his religious beliefs prompted immense guilt about hating others, especially a parent. Mixed feelings were illustrated by asking him to think of a time when his younger sibling did something that made him very angry. Gabriel was asked whether being extremely angry with his sibling meant he hated him. He responded spontaneously with laughter and realized it was possible to still love someone even if he disapproves of the person's behavior. Another technique that helped Gabriel cope when he became bothered by memories of his parents was more accurately labeling his feelings. The clinician helped Gabriel continue expanding his feelings vocabulary and encouraged him to use words other than hate and anger. He concluded that disappointment was a more appropriate term to describe his feelings about his parents, and this relabeling of his feelings reduced the intensity of much of his emotional reactions.

Conjoint Caregiver–Child Session

Gabriel was eager to share his narrative not only with Ms. R., but also with his new foster mother. Due to the level of preparation that had been done with Ms. R., the initial conjoint child–caregiver session was conducted with her. Gabriel no longer displayed avoidant reactions or emotional distress when thinking about his traumatic experiences and shared his narrative with Ms. R. without hesitation. They took turns in reading and, following the clinician's recommendations, Ms. R. was incredibly supportive and loving with Gabriel. With teary eyes, she expressed how proud she was of him and encouraged him to communicate with her if something similar to these traumas ever happened again. Given Gabriel's interest in sharing his narrative with his foster mother, the clinician briefed her on the events he would be discussing and encouraged her to display a supportive and accepting stance toward Gabriel during the conjoint session. Fortunately, the foster mother was a close friend of the family and was familiar with the events that had transpired, as she consoled Ms. R. numerous times in the past. Not surprisingly, when Gabriel's foster mother participated in the conjoint session, she was supportive and understanding.

Enhance Safety and Future Development

Safety planning with Gabriel included multiple sessions. First, a safety plan was developed, such as learning the phone number of his CPS caseworker and maintaining open communication with the adults in his life, especially Ms. R., who was in frequent contact with him. Safety planning also involved explaining to Gabriel the difference between "child and adult duties." For example, although his family was very proud of how brave he was to take on the responsibility of caring for his siblings during the previous episodes of neglect, the task of caring for other children was primarily for adults. He was praised for the work he did and was reminded that the best thing to do if a similar situation arose was to tell a trusting adult and seek help.

Near the end of treatment, Gabriel's foster mother began complaining about what she perceived to be "sexual acting out" from Gabriel. On multiple occasions Gabriel attempted to peek at his foster mother in the shower and as she was undressing in her bedroom. He performed the same behavior in relation to the foster mother's teenage daughter. The foster mother was bothered by the idea that Gabriel could be "fantasizing" about them, and that his behavior was immoral and a sign of sexual deviance. His foster mother believed Gabriel's acting out was related to his exposure to pornography that was part of his maltreatment history. Psychoeducation was presented to the foster mother by providing her with a fact sheet about sexual development and behavior in children, and assuring her that Gabriel's behavior was normal for his developmental level.

Nonetheless, these behaviors created significant distress for her, and she was uncertain how to respond. New treatment goals were developed, which involved establishing open communication about sexual behavior between Gabriel and his foster parents. In addition to discussing interpersonal boundaries and rules with Gabriel, the clinician and foster mother developed a behavior modification plan to correct the voyeuristic behavior. Despite the clinician's repeated suggestions that sexual psychoeducation be implemented with Gabriel, the foster parents resisted, invoking religious beliefs that such discussions were inappropriate. They also feared "further sexualizing" Gabriel. The clinician encouraged them to seek guidance on this issue from the religious leader at their church.

TREATMENT COMPLETION

TF-CBT treatment included a total of 18 sessions over 7 months. At the end of the intervention, neither Gabriel nor Ms. R. reported significant emotional or behavioral concerns. His foster mother completed a BASC-2 and TSCYC, and no significant elevations were noted. She denied he was experiencing any irritability, uncontrollable anger outbursts, sadness, or posttraumatic stress symptoms.

After the completion of TF-CBT, Gabriel continued in biweekly therapy. The foster parents' consultation with their religious leader resulted in a recommendation that Gabriel complete sexual psychoeducation with the clinician. Gabriel participated well in sessions with a new focus on sexual topics, and his foster mother reported that the behavior management plan was working well. Gabriel and his foster parents continued to work on these issues, and both learned ways to openly discuss sexual topics and behavior with each other. The foster parents helped Gabriel continue to implement the TF-CBT coping skills learned in treatment. Gabriel's treatment was complete. Approximately 3 months following treatment discharge, Ms. R. successfully petitioned for custody of the children. Gabriel returned to living with Ms. R. and was reunited with his siblings. There was no recurrence of emotional or behavioral problems.

COMMENTARY

This case study describes several all too common challenges to using TF-CBT in community service settings with multiproblem families. Most important, it illustrates how a clinician can develop creative solutions to meet those challenges effectively and deliver TF-CBT with an acceptable level of fidelity. Gabriel came to treatment not only with a history of exposure to multiple forms of abuse and neglect and with serious mental health problems as a result, but also a history of unsuccessful treatment. The child displayed serious avoidance reactions and an unsupportive grandmother buttressing them. And new stressful life events occurred during treatment. Collectively, these case characteristics may seriously hinder successful treatment. This case demonstrates that creativity, focusing on treatment goals, and clinician diligence and persistence are critical to successful outcomes. Several issues illustrate the challenges of this case and the creativity used as part of the therapy approach.

Intake Information

Gabriel presented with several problematic behaviors that often are signs of a serious trauma history. Anger outbursts, throwing objects, and irritability are common among children coming to mental health treatment, and frankly do not raise many cautions among experienced therapists. However, physical self-harm (head banging), animal cruelty, and stealing frequently signal a more guarded prognosis. Stealing is often associated with physical and emotional neglect, one of the most insidious forms of maltreatment that often results in persistent problems even when effective therapies are used.

Isolated animal cruelty can be the result of simple modeling behavior in a violent home, or it can be more cause for alarm if it has become a recurrent and pleasurable experience for the child. Physical self-harm is often used for immediate tension reduction and anxiety management, and it can be quite effective for that purpose for some children. Helping children progress from using self-harm to more adaptive coping methods, which may not have the immediate distraction and calming effect of physical self-harm, can be difficult. Therefore, this child clearly had some clinical challenges that were immediately evident based on the intake and assessment information.

Previous Therapy Experience

Traumatized children like Gabriel who previously participated in rather unstructured and lengthy therapy without meaningful success bring unique issues to the TF-CBT clinician. First, both the caregiver and the child now hold a certain view of what therapy is: unstructured; guided by the child; likely focused mostly on things that happened within the past week or so; composed almost exclusively of activities viewed as fun by the child; no "homework" or out-of-session practice activities; minimal involvement of the caregiver in the treatment process; little direct discussion of unpleasant or traumatic experiences, which are not shared with others; failure to really measure outcomes; and uncertainty about when treatment will end. Essentially, TF-CBT is the opposite, as Gabriel noted in the middle of therapy when he said TF-CBT was not as much fun as his prior therapy and there was a lot of work involved. Therefore, orienting the child and the caregiver to the process and elements of TF-CBT is even more critical with families that received different types of treatment in the past. In this case, understanding Gabriel's history, the clinician adapted to the situation and introduced some unstructured play time into the session routine to keep Gabriel engaged but maintained adherence to the TF-CBT model. This sort of clinical flexibility is crucial to continued engagement and treatment success.

Second, families completing unsuccessful therapy may be even more discouraged than the typical family coming to treatment. They may have little hope that any therapy can help, given their past experience. Inspiring hope that things will be better, a primary goal of the psychoeducation component of TF-CBT, can be more difficult with these families. TF-CBT clinicians need to be creative as they explain to families how this therapy is different from their past experiences and why it is likely to achieve positive results. This explanation needs to be done in a way that respects the previous therapist and the work the family did with him or her. Many children, like Gabriel, and their caregivers are very fond of their previous clinicians and may have enjoyed the therapy even though it did not reach the desired goals.

Avoidance

Few children are excited to come to therapy and talk about the details of the worst things that have happened in their lives. However, Gabriel seems to have had greater than average avoidance symptoms and problems approaching his trauma history. In this case, at least two contextual factors should be (and likely were) considered by the clinician. First, the grandmother's disdain of treatment and beliefs that prayer and spirituality should be used to manage suffering likely reinforced Gabriel's avoidance behavior. The clinician made an effort to engage the grandmother, but settled on Ms. R. as the supportive adult. However, any effort to reduce avoidance still must take into account the grandmother's views and her influence on Gabriel.

Second, the grandmother's views about therapy and how to manage suffering may not be hers alone. They may stem from common Latino/a cultural constructs, particularly the ideas of *machismo*, being strong, providing for, protecting and defending the family; *familismo*, keeping close to the family; and *marianismo*, being spiritually strong and enduring suffering in the image of the Virgin Mary (De Arellano, Danielson, & Felton, 2012). These views may be held by other family members, peers, and other individuals important to Gabriel. Cultural and community beliefs that support child avoidance are common among many groups. Clinicians should not assume that they are held by every family of a particular cultural heritage; rather, this should be assessed. In this case, attempts to engage the grandmother should assess and take into account, if necessary, the potentially larger cultural issues and beliefs that support the grandmother's attitudes about therapy for her grandson. Also in working with Gabriel, the potential influence on him of these and other cultural beliefs that can lead to greater avoidance should be assessed and accommodated in treatment as needed. Clinicians will need to creatively adapt therapy to reduce avoidance in a culturally competent way.

This clinician did a wonderful job of helping Gabriel think and talk about his trauma history beginning with the psychoeducation component. The technique of using third-party storytelling, either through books or other methods, is a common one to help avoidant children approach anxiety-producing memories, yet keep an emotional distance through a meta-position to the story. The clinician was able to engage the caregiver (but unfortunately not the grandmother) in this process to provide support for Gabriel as he struggled to talk about what he had experienced. Finally, the therapist encouraged gradual exposure throughout the PRAC components of TF-CBT to prepare the child for the trauma narrative. Although the child had some difficulties during the trauma narrative process, he successfully completed it. His success likely was the result of the early and ongoing gradual exposure used during all the earlier phases of treatment, coupled with the caregiver support fostered by the therapist.

Maintaining the Treatment Focus

At several critical points, the clinician easily could have been diverted from TF-CBT and moved in another therapeutic direction chasing the many emerging problems. Encountering *crises of the week* (or COWs) is common when treating children living in abusive and dysfunctional families. It is very easy to get sidetracked by these events and repeatedly alter the path of therapy to respond to each of them. Clinicians can find themselves changing course every few weeks as new incidents occur, meaning effective therapy is never done. In this case, the therapist was confronted with the grandparents losing their house, a school suspension, the removal of the child from his home, and placement in foster care. Any of these problems might have derailed Gabriel's trauma treatment. However, the clinician did an excellent job of acknowledging and managing each of the emerging difficulties, while maintaining the focus on trauma treatment. This process demonstrated the importance of continuing to focus on the treatment goals and exercising therapeutic discipline, diligence, and persistence in the trauma treatment. Sustaining treatment focus in the face of serious new events is not easy. Many COWs can be quite serious and appear to need immediate and ongoing attention and intervention. However, it is frequently the case that problem-solving the immediate situation and pushing forward with trauma treatment will have better results than launching in a new direction.

Summary

This case illustrates the importance of therapeutic creativity while maintaining treatment focus and adherence to the TF-CBT model. This clinician faced a case with many challenging elements and responded with purposeful adaptations. The clinician easily could have gotten sidetracked by the serious incidents that occurred during treatment. However, she kept her focus on the treatment goals, was able to manage the emerging difficulties, and helped this child and caregiver move successfully through the treatment.

REFERENCES

Briere, J. (2005). *Trauma Symptom Checklist for Young Children*. Odessa, FL: Psychological Assessment Resources.

De Arellano, M. A., Danielson, C. K., & Felton, J. W. (2012). Children of Latino descent: Culturally modified TF-CBT. In J. A. Cohen, A. P. Mannarino, & E. Deblinger

(Eds.), *Trauma-Focused CBT for children and adolescents: Treatment applications*. New York: Guilford Press.

Holmes, M. M. (2000). *A terrible thing happened*. Washington, DC: American Psychological Association.

Reynolds, C. R., & Kamphaus, R. W. (2004). *Behavior Assessment System for Children* (2nd ed.). Circle Pines, MN: AGS.

PART III

CHILD–PARENT PSYCHOTHERAPY (CPP)

6

Child–Parent Psychotherapy

An Overview

Mindy Kronenberg

$\mathbf{C}$hild–parent psychotherapy (CPP) is an evidence-based treatment for children from birth through age 5 and their caregivers. CPP was developed by Alicia Lieberman and Patricia Van Horn for children exposed to domestic violence (2005) and for children who experienced the death of a primary caregiver (Lieberman, Compton, Van Horn, & Ghosh Ippen, 2003). CPP also has been described as an effective treatment for children with a variety of traumatic stressors as well as normative life stressors and mental health issues (Lieberman & Van Horn, 2008). The current chapter provides an overview of CPP as a treatment for trauma-exposed children and their caregivers.

THEORETICAL RATIONALE

CPP embraces multiple theoretical perspectives to capture the full complexity of human experience. CPP draws primarily from attachment, psychoanalytic, and trauma theories and includes intervention strategies from cognitive-behavioral and social learning theories. In addition, CPP recognizes the overarching necessity of viewing individuals within sociocultural and developmental frameworks (Lieberman & Van Horn, 2005, 2008).

Attachment and Trauma Theories

CPP is first and foremost a relationship-based intervention that utilizes the caregiver–child relationship to promote a child's optimal mental health and development. The quality of the relationship is associated with the child's attachment, defined as the emotional bond between a specific caregiver and child (Bowlby, 1969). Ideally, a caregiver responds to a child's behaviors in a sensitive and responsive manner, and the child is able to develop a "secure attachment." The child then utilizes that caregiver as a "secure base" for exploring the world and providing a sense of safety and security in times of distress (Ainsworth, Blehar, Waters, & Wall, 1978). CPP follows the attachment theory premise that the safety of the caregiving relationship is the foundation that enables appropriate social, emotional, and cognitive development. Within this early attachment relationship, a child also forms "internal working models" that serve as templates for understanding and establishing expectations about the world, the self, and others (Bowlby, 1969).

It is important to note the interplay between attachment and trauma theories (Lieberman, 2004). Infants do not possess adequate physiological and emotional regulation skills to cope with traumatic events. Therefore, the deleterious effects of trauma may adversely affect the development of the child's neurological system as well as social, emotional, and cognitive skills (Van der Kolk, 2005). Furthermore, the experience of trauma affects the child's internal working model in such a way that the child no longer views the world as a safe place; rather, the child expects that the world is dangerous and that little or no protection is available (Pynoos, Steinberg, Ornitz, & Goenjian, 1997).

Secure attachment can buffer the impact of trauma; however, trauma can disrupt attachment (Cassidy & Mohr, 2001). When the attachment figure is either a perpetrator of violence or is unable to protect the child from external traumatic forces, that individual may lose the role of the child's protective shield (Freud, 1926/1959). This situation creates a frightening dilemma for the child. From an attachment perspective, the child has an innate tendency to seek safety from an attachment figure; however, from a trauma perspective, the attachment figure may remind the child of the trauma, which results in the child's responding with avoidance, fear, and/or confusion (Lieberman, 2004; Pynoos, Steinberg, & Piacentini, 1999).

Psychoanalytic Theory

Along with attachment theory, psychoanalytic theory guides CPP's formulation of the impact of trauma and provides a rationale explaining the repetition of maltreatment across generations. Psychoanalytic theory is based on several basic principles, including the understanding that experiences from the past affect how an individual thinks, feels, and behaves in the present, and that behavior is affected by factors outside of conscious awareness. CPP's psychoanalytic roots may best be described by acknowledging the contributions of Selma Fraiberg (1980), who developed infant–parent psychotherapy (IPP), the precursor of CPP. Both IPP (an intervention for children from birth through age 3 and their caregivers) and CPP (which extends the age range through 5 years of age) emphasize the effects of caregivers' attributions on children's developing sense of self.

Fraiberg, Adelson, and Shapiro (1975) described caregivers' negative attributions about their children's behaviors as being based on the caregivers' internal working models, which were formed during their own, often traumatic, childhoods. They referred to these traumatic internal working models' recurrence in the present as "ghosts in the nursery." For example, a mother with her own history of physical abuse may view her baby's crying as proof that the baby is angry and wants to hurt her. The mother may, in turn, respond harshly toward the baby. Similarly, a father with a history of abandonment may interpret his toddler's exploration of the environment as a lack of interest in their relationship and respond by further disengaging from the toddler. In both of these examples, the children may be directly negatively affected by their caregivers' behaviors and also internalize their caregivers' beliefs, thereby developing their own maladaptive internal working models. In this manner, parenting styles, ways of relating, and even maltreatment may be passed from parent to child and sometimes on to the child's children. This cycle is referred to as the "intergenerational transmission of trauma" (Lieberman, 2004; Schechter & Willheim, 2009).

TREATMENT THEMES

CPP clinicians maintain an awareness that behavior has meaning and that trauma may affect how an individual behaves and perceives others. CPP clinicians seek to understand the totality of the caregiver's and child's experiences and recognize the need to view individuals within the contexts of attachment, trauma, development, and culture. Throughout treatment, the clinician is responsive to both the caregiver's and child's emotional processes (including affect regulation), supportive of a physically and emotionally safe caregiver–child relationship, and mindful of the importance of directly addressing traumatic experiences, reminders, and symptoms during treatment (Ghosh Ippen, Van Horn, & Lieberman, 2012).

Focus on the Caregiver–Child Relationship

CPP focuses on the caregiver–child relationship and seeks to strengthen this relationship to promote optimal child development. When a caregiver and child present for CPP, the relationship is frequently beset by problems and tainted by negative patterns of interaction. The child may display either internalizing or externalizing symptoms, and the caregiver may behave harshly toward, ignore, or reject the child. These negative patterns of relating often reflect the damaging impact of trauma on caregivers' and children's perceptions of each other.

CPP targets these trauma-related perceptions for change by having the clinician adopt the role of translator between caregiver and child. For example, when a caregiver seeks treatment to reduce a child's "bad" or "mean" behavior, the clinician begins by working with the caregiver to understand the underlying meaning of the behavior (e.g., developmentally appropriate, dysregulation following a trauma, modeling of negative adult or peer behaviors). Similarly, if the child views a safe caregiver who sets appropriate limits as "mean" or "scary," the clinician, along with the caregiver, helps the child recognize the caregiver as a source of protection. As the members of the dyad respond to each other in a more realistic and positive manner, they begin to engage in new, more adaptive patterns of relating (Lieberman & Van Horn, 2005, 2008).

Emphasis on Reflective Capacity

In order to address the symptoms or relational problems that dyads present in treatment, the clinician must understand both the caregiver's and the child's internal working models that inherently guide how they perceive the world and respond to others. Therefore, reflective functioning, or the ability to think about the thoughts and feelings of the self and others (Fonagy, Steele, Steele, Moran, & Higgitt, 1991), is a cornerstone of CPP and a defining characteristic of skilled CPP clinicians. Clinicians with highly developed reflective capacities are aware of their emotional reactions and the effects that their emotional states may have on others. Reflective capacity ensures that clinicians consider others' perspectives and reflect on the meanings of their behaviors. In the context of trauma work, reflective capacity is necessary in order for clinicians to remain emotionally available and know when they need to regulate their own cognitive, emotional, and physiological responses to the traumatic material that dyads bring to therapy.

Reflective capacity is also facilitated when clinicians engage with colleagues or supervisors who support them in reflecting on the therapeutic process. The support that clinicians receive is viewed as necessary; thus, to achieve CPP fidelity, obtaining reflective supervision or consultation is required (Ghosh Ippen et al., 2012). Supervision and/or consultation prevents burnout and secondary traumatic stress (Figley, 2002) and enables clinicians to more effectively treat families (see Sommer & Spielman, Chapter 8, this volume, for a case study jointly written by a clinician and supervisor).

PROGRAM COMPONENTS AND CHARACTERISTICS

A basic tenet of trauma treatment is that humans strive to create structure and gain a sense of safety and control in a world that is often unpredictable. CPP embraces the dialect of the need for predictability in an unpredictable world and accepts that treatment cannot always unfold in a prescribed manner. CPP was designed as a flexible approach in which the clinician follows the needs of the family, rather than a series of treatment steps. CPP facilitates predictability by creating a consistent and safe therapeutic environment in which healthy development and caregiver–child interactions are supported (Lieberman & Van Horn, 2005, 2008).

Treatment Goals

Treatment is shaped by the overarching goal of supporting normal development in a child whose developmental trajectory has been affected by trauma. The clinician achieves this overarching goal by focusing on several subgoals (Lieberman & Van Horn, 2005).

1. Increase ability to regulate emotions.
2. Increase ability to recognize and understand feelings associated with bodily sensations.

These subgoals seek to establish or restore capacities that are generally developed in the context of nurturing early childhood relationships and may be derailed by the trauma.

3. Break negative cycles of interaction and build mutually satisfying caregiver–child relationships based on understanding.

This subgoal reflects the importance of attachment theory in CPP and addresses relational problems that may result from trauma.

4. Normalize traumatic responses.
5. Increase ability to respond realistically to threat.
6. Increase ability to differentiate remembering from reexperiencing.
7. Place the traumatic experience in perspective so that the trauma is integrated as a part of the child's life and the dyad's experience.

These subgoals encourage the caregiver and child to directly address trauma-related symptoms so they can focus on present and future-oriented goals.

Core Competencies

The flexibility of CPP is a strength of the model in that it allows the clinician to follow the dyad's needs while moving toward treatment goals. However, the flexibility also lends itself to a complex approach that requires clinicians to have strong foundational knowledge and skills in order to confidently and adeptly implement the model. Core knowledge areas include child and adult development and psychopathology as well as an understanding of sociocultural influences on individual functioning. Furthermore, a clinician must have the following abilities: to observe behavior, to collaborate with multiple service systems, to translate between caregivers' and children's experiences, and to maintain reflective functioning. Each of these areas represents an overarching value of CPP (Van Horn & Lieberman, 2010).

Treatment Process

CPP was manualized as a 12-month intervention with weekly sessions (Lieberman & Van Horn, 2005). Depending on the needs of the family, CPP may be shorter (see Sommer & Spielman, Chapter 8, this volume) or longer (see Many, Chapter 7, this volume). A hallmark of CPP is the dyadic nature of the intervention in which both caregiver and child are in the room; however, the flexibility of CPP allows for variations in this process. There are times when individual child or caregiver sessions may be required. For example, an individual session with a caregiver may be necessary to discuss the caregiver's trauma history. There are other times when multiple caregivers or multiple children are involved in CPP. When an exception is made and the caregiver or child is seen alone, the therapeutic goal of strengthening the attachment relationship remains primary. Similarly, when CPP is conducted with multiple members of the family in the room, the caregiver–child relationship, rather than the family system, remains the target of intervention (Lieberman & Van Horn, 2008).

When intervening, the clinician chooses interventions that strengthen the caregiver–child relationship and empower the caregiver to intervene on behalf of the child. The clinician avoids usurping the caregiver's role with the child or taking on the role of the expert whose parenting skills the caregiver is encouraged to model. Rather, the clinician maintains a curious and collaborative stance and helps the caregiver develop a protective and supportive parenting style (Van Horn & Lieberman, 2010).

Assessment, Engagement, and Introducing the Child to CPP

Treatment begins with a comprehensive assessment that provides the foundation for case conceptualization and treatment planning. The assessment is conducted over three to five 45-minute sessions during which the clinician first meets individually with the caregiver and then observes the caregiver–child interaction (Zero to Three, 2005). Assessment includes evaluation of both the caregiver's and child's trauma histories and symptomatology. The clinician begins to understand the experiences of each member of the dyad, and how these experiences affect the caregiver's and child's internal working models, and to identify potential trauma triggers. The clinician also attends to the dyad's positive experiences in order to capitalize on the strengths the dyad brings to treatment. While conducting the assessment, the clinician explains that the caregiver will be an active participant in treatment planning and throughout the intervention.

The assessment period sets the stage for an intervention in which the internal worlds of both the caregiver and child are valued and explored. The clinician provides an overview of treatment, including an explanation of trauma responses, trauma reminders, and the impact of the caregiver's own childhood experiences on parenting. During this process, the clinician learns about the caregiver's feelings regarding the use of play as a therapeutic modality, the caregiver's acceptance of open discussions of trauma, and the caregiver's understanding of the impact of trauma on the child (Ghosh Ippen et al., 2012; Lieberman & Van Horn, 2008). By the end of assessment, the caregiver and clinician come to an agreement about how to introduce CPP and provide the child with a clear reason for therapy. This explanation acknowledges the connection between the child's symptoms and the child's traumatic experiences, gives the child permission to talk openly about memories of and feelings about the trauma, and assures the child that symptom reduction can occur (Van Horn & Lieberman, 2010).

Intervention

When intervening with a family, ensuring physical and emotional safety is always the first priority. If these needs reemerge during the course of treatment, they again take priority. After helping to establish basic needs, the clinician utilizes simple interventions before more complex interventions are employed. Simple interventions, such as providing developmental guidance about age-appropriate behavior, may change the caregiver's maladaptive working models and lead to more positive caregiver–child interactions. When simple interventions are not effective, the clinician's goal is to understand and address barriers that impede treatment progress (Lieberman & Van Horn, 2005, 2008).

In deciding when and how to intervene, the clinician uses "ports of entry" (Stern, 1995), opportunities to engage with the caregiver and/or child in order to further therapeutic progress. Ports of entry are chosen based on the needs, the therapeutic goals, and the readiness of the dyad to benefit from the intervention. Common ports of entry include the caregiver's or child's behavior; the caregiver–child interaction; the caregiver's or child's representations of the self or the other; and the relationship between the clinician, caregiver, and child. As long as the clinician adheres to the model's basic principles, CPP does not limit the types of interventions that may be utilized at any given port of entry. The following techniques are commonly used in CPP (Lieberman & Van Horn, 2005, 2008):

Crisis Intervention/Case Management/Concrete Assistance. Interventions that help a family obtain basic needs such as food, housing, and medical care honor the belief that physical needs and safety issues must first be addressed before a dyad can fully engage in an intervention focused on social or emotional issues (Maslow, 1943). CPP recognizes that in order for psychotherapy to have a generalized impact, it must address not only the caregiver and child, but also community agencies and systems that interact with the family. CPP clinicians may coordinate with schools, courts, primary care offices, or any other system. In this manner, the clinician helps a caregiver successfully navigate systems that may be perceived as frightening or overwhelming (see Many, Chapter 7, and Sommer & Spielman, Chapter 8, this volume, for examples of CPP in the context of child welfare and substance use treatment).

Modeling Protective Behavior. Clinicians use this intervention when a caregiver or child is behaving in an unsafe manner. For example, a clinician would model protective behavior when a child stands or climbs on unstable furniture. If the caregiver does not recognize that the child may be hurt, the clinician would consider verbalizing the concerns to the caregiver. If the child is about to fall and the caregiver does not react, the clinician would physically help the child regain safety. Clinicians also model protective behavior in situations relevant to aspects of daily living that involve the overall safety of the family. For example, a clinician may decline to conduct home visits when an abusive partner is in the house. When interventions such as these occur, the clinician provides an explanation and remains mindful of and encourages discussion about the caregiver's response. The goal of modeling protective behavior is to help the caregiver and child respond realistically to threat and for the caregiver to return to the protective role (Lieberman & Van Horn, 2005, 2008).

Promoting Developmental Progress through Play, Physical Contact, and Language. The use of language, play, and nurturing physical contact between caregiver and child provide opportunities for the child to make sense of the world and learn to engage in socially appropriate behaviors and relationships. Therapy sessions offer a dedicated time, with a physically safe space and emotionally safe environment, in which a caregiver and child can learn about each other and enjoy being together. The clinician engages with both members of the dyad, joins their interaction, and facilitates the caregiver and child's communication about both positive and negative experiences.

Interactive symbolic play helps young children communicate feelings and experiences. Therefore, the clinician ensures that a variety of toys to support this play are available (e.g., human, animal, and vehicle figurines; pretend food and dishes). As children develop verbal skills, encouraging the verbal expression of feelings becomes increasingly important in order for children to successfully cope with emotions and express needs. Furthermore, appropriate physical displays of affection between caregivers and children are always important in expressing nurturing, caring, and love. In addition to supporting caregiver–child communication, these types of interactions also promote physical, behavioral, and emotional regulation. For example, bubbles may aid in relaxation through breathing, the sensory comfort of sand may help a child communicate through sand tray toys, and a soft ball may be rhythmically rolled between child and caregiver to promote mutually attuned engagement. As a dyad progresses in therapy, they are able to achieve healthy patterns of interaction independently and no longer require the clinician's guidance (Lieberman & Van Horn, 2005, 2008).

Addressing Trauma Reminders. Throughout treatment, the clinician, caregiver, and child address behaviors that result from trauma reminders. The clinician provides developmental guidance to help both the caregiver and child notice when the child's behavior is based on a trauma response and helps both members of the dyad develop skills for coping with trauma-related symptoms. A common theme of trauma treatments and a mechanism to reduce trauma-related symptoms is the development of a trauma narrative (cf. Cohen, Mannarino, & Deblinger, 2006). The narrative a caregiver and child create about their trauma experiences is a component of CPP; however, given the developmental phase of children who participate in CPP, narratives are generally not presented as a discrete event or product. Infants and young children often create narratives through their bodies or through behavior in play. For example, an infant who begins treatment by clinging to her mother without being able to soothe and ends treatment by actively exploring the toys and returning to her mother for comfort when distressed, has created a narrative. She used her body, affect, and behavior to communicate her perspective that at first she could not regulate her fear; however, by the end of treatment, she communicated that she viewed the world as an exciting place and her mother as an individual who could help her regulate both positive and negative emotions. The clinician's role here may be described as "behavior translator" when reflecting on the changes in the child's behavior with the caregiver.

Preschool-age children may use play in order to construct a trauma narrative. With the consent of the caregiver, the clinician ensures the availability of toys (e.g., emergency vehicles, handcuffs)—assuming they are not overstimulating as trauma reminders— to help the child communicate about traumatic experiences. It is important that a variety of toys be available and that the child be allowed to choose the toys with which to play. There is no preset phase of the treatment process when the child is expected to create a trauma narrative. However, as the child feels an increased sense of safety in the caregiver's presence, the child, with the support of the caregiver and clinician, is able to spontaneously communicate about traumatic experiences and feelings (Lieberman & Van Horn, 2005, 2008).

Providing Emotional Support. In CPP, the relationship between the clinician and the caregiver has particular significance. Given that it is the caregiver, rather than the clinician, who supports the child's development, the caregiver must have the capacity to offer this support. However, many caregivers who present to treatment lack social support as well as a model of an emotionally supportive caregiver from childhood. Therefore, the clinician provides emotional support to the caregiver. This support is offered in many ways including providing encouragement and hope, helping the caregiver self-regulate when distressed, and responding to the caregiver in a reflective manner. Ideally, a parallel process occurs and, as the caregiver feels supported by the clinician, the caregiver is better able to support the child. With the supportive caregiver–child relationship in place, the caregiver and child are better able to utilize therapy sessions to address trauma responses and other symptoms (Lieberman & Van Horn, 2005, 2008).

Offering Unstructured, Reflective Developmental Guidance. Clinicians provide information when a caregiver's lack of understanding about issues related to child development, parenting, or the impact of trauma is associated with problems in the dyad. In CPP, developmental guidance is not based on a curriculum; rather, the content and timing are based on the needs of the caregiver and child. Furthermore, the clinician tailors the information to the developmental stage, sociocultural context, and trauma history of the family. Information is generally provided in a conversational manner during which the clinician asks about the caregiver's past and current experiences related to the topic. The unstructured nature of developmental guidance is intended to support the caregiver's development of reflective capacity. With both increased knowledge and increased reflective capacity, the caregiver is able to think about the internal world of the child, to understand the meaning of the child's behavior, and to gain increased empathy for the child (Lieberman & Van Horn, 2005, 2008).

When providing developmental guidance, the clinician often seeks the caregiver's feedback to ascertain the caregiver's acquisition of the information and to determine whether the information needs to be further tailored to the family or delivered in a different manner. "Speaking for baby" is an intervention that may be employed when a caregiver has difficulty accepting information presented directly (Carter, Osofsky, & Hann, 1991). In this intervention, the clinician uses the child's figurative voice to convey information. For example, a caregiver who fears that he will spoil his infant daughter if he picks her up when she cries may respond more effectively when a clinician speaks for the baby by saying, "Daddy, I love it when you hold me; I learn how to stop crying." During this type of intervention, even though the caregiver knows that a clinician is speaking, the caregiver still responds to the child as if the child has spoken. Thus the caregiver has a chance to practice hearing the child's needs and responding directly to them, rather than learning how to be responsive based on psychoeducation delivered in a didactic format.

Insight-Oriented Interpretation. Insight-oriented interventions are often used to address "ghosts in the nursery" (Fraiberg et al., 1975). To promote insight, the clinician asks questions, notices patterns, and reflects with the caregiver about past and present experiences. Over time and through reflective discussion, the caregiver recognizes when current negative patterns of interactions with a child are based on past childhood experiences, rather than present circumstances. When caregivers are able to think about their own childhood and remember painful experiences, they may be able to remember how it felt to be a child. When this occurs, caregivers are able to identify with and gain empathy for their own children and, in this manner, break the cycle of intergenerational transmission of trauma (Lieberman & Van Horn, 2005, 2008).

The development of positive caregiving relationships is supported not only by decreasing the repetition of negative patterns of parenting ("ghosts") but also by encouraging caregivers to remember and assimilate positive experiences from their own childhoods ("angels") into their current parenting practices (Lieberman, Padrón, Van Horn, & Harris, 2005). As caregivers are able to link past and present and recognize patterns they do not want to repeat, they are able to remember positive experiences and traditions that they would like to pass on to their children (Lieberman & Van Horn, 2008).

Termination

Treatment termination is planned jointly between the clinician and caregiver. Based on a 52-week model of CPP, the termination phase occurs during the last 3 months of treatment (Lieberman & Van Horn, 2005). The length of time devoted to termination highlights its importance. The end of treatment may represent a significant loss for the family, including the loss of stability afforded by the treatment process and the loss of the relationship with the clinician. During the termination phase, the clinician works to provide a new model of transition, helping the caregiver and child understand that all relationships need not end abruptly or traumatically. Thus the termination process focuses on differentiating the loss of the therapeutic relationship from previous traumatic losses the family experienced. Direct discussion of termination begins earlier with caregivers and later with children (approximately 1 month prior to the end of treatment), owing to their developmental experience of time (Ghosh Ippen et al., 2012). The clinician, caregiver, and child may discuss what was internalized from the therapeutic relationship, and the clinician may assure the caregiver and child that, even though the relationship is ending, the clinician will continue to hold them in mind (Lieberman & Van Horn 2005, 2008).

RESEARCH EVIDENCE FOR CPP

CPP is listed as an evidence-based treatment on the Substance Abuse and Mental Health Services Administration's (SAMHSA) National Registry of Evidence-Based Programs and Practices based on the results of five randomized controlled trials. This research was conducted by the CPP developers as well as by independent researchers.

Child Outcomes

Among a sample of preschool-age children who were exposed to marital violence, CPP was associated with reductions in posttraumatic stress symptoms, behavioral symptoms, and posttraumatic stress disorder (PTSD) diagnoses (Lieberman, Van Horn, & Ghosh Ippen, 2005). Furthermore, the improvements in behavioral functioning were maintained at a 6-month follow-up (Lieberman, Ghosh Ippen, & Van Horn, 2006). This sample was further studied to examine the efficacy of CPP among children who experienced multiple (four or more) traumas/stressors. Results suggested that CPP was particularly beneficial for this group and was linked to reductions in posttraumatic stress symptoms, behavioral symptoms, and depression, as well as PTSD and other comorbid diagnoses. These improvements also were maintained when measured at a 6-month follow-up (Ghosh Ippen, Harris, Van Horn, & Lieberman, 2011).

Caregiver Outcomes

Although the primary goal of CPP is to improve child functioning, caregivers who participate in CPP also benefit from the intervention. In the study described above examining preschool-age children, mothers in both the CPP and active control groups showed declines in levels of overall distress. However, only mothers in the CPP group had significantly decreased levels of PTSD avoidance symptoms following treatment (Lieberman et al., 2005). At the 6-month follow-up, CPP was associated with maintained reductions in the caregiver's overall level of distress (Lieberman et al., 2006). Furthermore, the mothers of the preschool-age children who experienced multiple traumas/stressors also benefited from CPP, as evidenced by reduced symptoms of PTSD and depression; these reductions were maintained at a 6-month follow-up (Ghosh Ippen et al., 2011).

Relational Outcomes

Researchers have utilized both caregiver report and clinical observation to demonstrate that CPP is linked to increased attachment security among young children (Cicchetti, Toth, & Rogosch, 1999; Toth, Rogosch, & Cicchetti, 2006). For instance, in one study, infants who received CPP displayed decreased avoidance, resistance, and anger toward their caregivers, and caregivers were noted to display increased empathy and engagement with their children (Lieberman, Weston, & Pawl, 1991).

Given that attachment and trauma affect how children perceive themselves and others, preschoolers' mental representations were utilized as an outcome measure in another CPP outcome study (Toth, Maughan, Manly, Spagnola, & Cicchetti, 2002). In this sample, CPP was associated with reductions in children's negative representations of themselves. Furthermore, increases in children's positive expectations of the mother–child relationship and decreases in maladaptive maternal representations were observed in children after participation in CPP. Although noticeable changes in these areas also were observed among children who received other interventions (active controls), children in the CPP group displayed the largest improvements in these areas.

CULTURAL CONSIDERATIONS

The research described provides support for the efficacy of CPP with diverse populations. CPP studies have included a trial with Latina immigrant mothers (Lieberman et al. 1991), a trial in which the majority of participants were of mixed ethnic (mostly Latino and white) or Latino decent (Lieberman et al., 2005), and trials with samples that were primarily African American (Toth et al., 2002) or white (Cicchetti et al., 1999; Toth et al. 2006). CPP research participants also vary regarding socioeconomic status. Mothers in one study had an average of 9.42 years of education, and 71.4% of the mothers were unemployed (Lieberman et al., 1991). In another study with caregivers on the other end of the socioeconomic spectrum, 54.5% of the mothers graduated college or held graduate degrees (Toth et al., 2006).

CPP's flexible approach allows for the cultural values of each dyad to play integral roles in determining the process of treatment. Although cultural competence is always of primary importance when using any intervention, fidelity to the CPP protocol requires that clinicians attend to a family's cultural beliefs; be aware of their own cultural biases; and understand families in terms of their cultural, ecological, and historical context (Ghosh Ippen et al., 2012). This attention to culture begins during the assessment when the clinician encourages open dialogue regarding sociocultural issues, asks questions regarding the dyad's cultural background and socioeconomic status, and obtains information regarding how these factors affect the caregiver's parenting style. Culture shapes all aspects of the intervention (Lewis & Ghosh Ippen, 2004). For example, playing with toys is a commonly used intervention modality. If, however, due to cultural issues or other factors, a caregiver is not comfortable with play, the clinician should be flexible in helping the caregiver find other ways to communicate and share enjoyable moments with the child.

CPP clinicians make efforts to ensure that socioeconomic and sociocultural barriers do not prohibit dyads from obtaining services. CPP was originally designed as a home visiting model, which allows increased access to services. CPP has been successfully integrated into pediatric primary care settings (Renschler, Lieberman, Dimmler, & Harris, 2013) and is regularly used in collaboration with child welfare systems (Osofsky et al., 2007; Van Horn et al., 2012). When issues related to immigration are present, concrete assistance, such as connecting an individual to an immigration attorney, may be necessary (Reyes & Lieberman, 2012).

In addition to individual intervention, CPP recognizes the importance of "supraclinical interventions" that address issues such as poverty, discrimination, disparities in access to mental health services, and the disproportionate number of young children exposed to trauma. "Supraclinical interventions," such as advocacy and public policy work, are necessary to create safe communities in which CPP can be truly effective (Harris, Lieberman, & Marans, 2007; Lieberman, Chu, Van Horn, & Harris, 2011).

TRAINING PROGRAMS AND RESOURCES

Clinicians are required to hold a master's degree to receive training in CPP. Training may be achieved in two ways: clinicians may either complete a predoctoral internship or postdoctoral fellowship that is certified to train

CPP clinicians or complete an 18-month training program based on the National Child Traumatic Stress Network's learning collaborative model. In order to promote model sustainability within an agency, learning collaboratives require clinicians, supervisors, and leaders to participate in the training and learn the model together. Trainings must be conducted by a trainer who is approved by the CPP development team. As of this volume's publication date, requirements for successful completion include (1) reading the treatment manuals (Lieberman & Van Horn, 2005, 2008); (2) attending three in-person trainings (an initial 3-day training and two follow-up 2-day trainings); (3) participating in and presenting cases during twice-monthly conference calls conducted by a CPP trainer; (4) participating in weekly reflective supervision; (5) carrying four cases, with at least one case lasting 11 sessions, during the 18-month training period; and (6) completing fidelity measures (Ghosh Ippen et al., 2012; Van Horn et al., 2012).

CONCLUSIONS

CPP is a relationship-based, trauma-informed intervention for children from birth through age 5 and their caregivers. The primary goal of CPP is to facilitate a child's return to a normal developmental trajectory following trauma. Research conducted with dyads of diverse ethnic and socioeconomic backgrounds demonstrates that CPP is associated with reductions in both caregiver and child symptomatology and increases in positive relational outcomes. This dyadic mode of intervention promotes protective and supportive caregiver–child relationships, thereby providing young children with the necessary foundation for optimal development.

SUGGESTED RESOURCES

Books

- Lieberman, A. F., Compton, N. C., Van Horn, P., & Ghosh Ippen, C. (2003). *Losing a parent to death in the early years: Guidelines for the treatment of traumatic bereavement in infancy.* Washington, DC: Zero to Three Press.

- Lieberman, A. F., & Van Horn, P. (2005). *Don't hit my mommy!: A manual for child–parent psychotherapy with young witnesses of family violence.* Washington, DC: Zero to Three Press.

- Lieberman, A. F., & Van Horn, P. (2008). *Psychotherapy with infants and young children: Repairing the effects of stress and trauma on early attachment.* New York: Guilford Press.

Websites

- National Child Traumatic Stress Network (description of CPP)
  www.nctsn.org/sites/default/files/assets/pdfs/cpp_general.pdf

- National Child Traumatic Stress Network (CPP culture-specific information)
  www.nctsnet.org/nctsn_assets/pdfs/promising_practices/CPP_Culture%20_7-13-07.pdf

- Substance Abuse and Mental Health Services Administration's National Registry of Evidence-Based Programs and Practices
  www.nrepp.samhsa.gov/ViewIntervention.aspx?id=194

- University of California, San Francisco, Child Trauma Research Program
  http://psych.ucsf.edu/research.aspx?id=1554

REFERENCES

Ainsworth, M. D. S., Blehar, M. C., Waters, E., & Wall, S. (1978). Patterns of attachment: A psychological study of the strange situation. Hillsdale: Erlbaum.

Bowlby, J. (1969). Attachment and loss: Vol. 1. Attachment. New York: Basic Books.

Carter, S. L., Osofsky, J. D., & Hann, D. M. (1991). Speaking for the baby: A therapeutic intervention with adolescent mothers and their infants. Infant Mental Health Journal, 12, 291–301.

Cassidy, J., & Mohr, J. J. (2001). Unsolvable fear, trauma, and psychopathology: Theory, research, and clinical considerations related to disorganized attachment across the life span. Clinical Psychology: Science and Practice, 8, 275–298.

Cohen, J. A., Mannarino, A. P., & Deblinger, E. (2006). Treating trauma and traumatic grief in children and adolescents. New York: Guilford Press.

Cicchetti, D., Rogosch, F.A., & Toth, S.L. (2006). Fostering secure attachment in infants in maltreating families through preventative interventions. Development and Psychopathology, 18, 623–650.

Cicchetti, D., Toth, S. L., & Rogosch, F. A. (1999). The efficacy of toddler–parent psychotherapy to increase attachment security in offspring of depressed mothers. Attachment and Human Development, 1, 34–66.

Figley, C. R. (2002). Compassion fatigue: Psychotherapists' chronic lack of self care. Journal of Clinical Psychology, 58, 1433–1441.

Fonagy, P., Steele, M., Steele, H., Moran, G. S., & Higgitt, A. C. (1991). The capacity for understanding mental states: The reflective self in parent and child and its significance for security of attachment. Infant Mental Health Journal, 12, 201–218.

Fraiberg, S. (1980). Clinical studies in infant mental health. New York: Basic Books.

Fraiberg, S., Adelson, E., & Shapiro, V. (1975). Ghosts in the nursery: A psychoanalytic approach to the problems of impaired infant–mother relationships. Journal of the American Academy of Child Psychiatry, 14, 387–421.

Freud, S. (1959). Inhibitions, symptoms and anxiety. In J. Strachey (Ed. & Trans.), The standard edition of the complete psychological works of Sigmund Freud. London: Hogarth Press. (Original published 1926)

Ghosh Ippen, C., Harris, W. W., Van Horn, P., & Lieberman, A. F. (2011). Traumatic and stressful events in early childhood: Can treatment help those at highest risk? *Child Abuse and Neglect, 35,* 504–513.

Ghosh Ippen, C., Van Horn, P., & Lieberman, A. F. (2012). *The CPP Fidelity Assessment Toolkit.* Unpublished measure.

Harris, W. W., Lieberman, A. F., & Marans, S. (2007). In the best interests of society. *Journal of Child Psychology and Psychiatry, 48,* 392–411.

Lewis, M. L., & Ghosh Ippen, C. G. (2004). Rainbows of tears, souls full of hope: Cultural issues related to young children and trauma. In J. D. Osofsky (Ed.), *Young children and trauma: Intervention and treatment.* New York: Guilford Press.

Lieberman, A. F. (2004). Traumatic stress and quality of attachment: Reality and internalization in disorders of infant mental health. *Infant Mental Health Journal, 25,* 336–351.

Lieberman, A. F., Chu, A., Van Horn, P., & Harris, W. W. (2011). Trauma in early childhood: Empirical evidence and clinical implications. *Development and Psychopathology, 23,* 397–410.

Lieberman, A. F., Compton, N. C., Van Horn, P., & Ghosh Ippen, C. (2003). *Losing a parent to death in the early years: Guidelines for the treatment of traumatic bereavement in infancy.* Washington, DC: Zero to Three Press.

Lieberman, A. F., Ghosh Ippen, C., & Van Horn, P. (2006). Child-parent psychotherapy: 6-month follow-up of a randomized controlled trial. *Journal of the American Academy of Child and Adolescent Psychiatry, 45,* 913–918.

Lieberman, A. F., Padrón, E., Van Horn, P., & Harris, W. W. (2005). Angels in the nursery: The intergenerational transmission of benevolent parental influences. *Infant Mental Health Journal, 26,* 504–520.

Lieberman, A. F., & Van Horn, P. (2005). *Don't hit my mommy!: A manual for child–parent psychotherapy with young witnesses of family violence.* Washington, DC: Zero to Three Press.

Lieberman, A. F., & Van Horn, P. (2008). *Psychotherapy with infants and young children: Repairing the effects of stress and trauma on early attachment.* New York: Guilford Press.

Lieberman, A. F., Van Horn, P., & Ghosh Ippen, C. (2005). Toward evidence-based treatment: Child-parent psychotherapy with preschoolers exposed to marital violence. *Journal of the American Academy of Child and Adolescent Psychiatry, 44,* 1241–1248.

Lieberman, A. F., Weston, D. R., & Pawl, J. H. (1991). Preventive intervention and outcome with anxiously attached dyads. *Child Development, 62,* 199–209.

Maslow, A. H. (1943). A theory of human motivation. *Psychological Review, 50,* 370–396.

Osofsky, J. D., Kronenberg, M., Hammer, J. H., Lederman, J. C., Katz, L., Adams, S., et al. (2007). The development and evaluation of the intervention model for the Florida Infant Mental Health Pilot Program. *Infant Mental Health Journal, 28,* 259–280.

Pynoos, R. S., Steinberg, A. M., Ornitz, E. M., & Goenjian, A. K. (1997). Issues in the developmental neurobiology of traumatic stress. *Annals of the New York Academy of Sciences, 821,* 176–193

Pynoos, R. S., Steinberg, A. M., & Piacentini, J. C. (1999). A developmental psychopathology model of childhood traumatic stress and intersection with anxiety disorders. *Biological Psychiatry, 46,* 1542–1554.

Renschler, T. S., Lieberman, A. F., Dimmler, M. H., & Harris, N. B. (2013). Trauma-focused Child-parent psychotherapy in a community pediatric clinic: A cross-disciplinary collaboration. In J. E. Bettman & D. D. Friedman (Eds.), *Attachment-based clinical work with children and adolescents*. New York: Springer.

Reyes, V. & Lieberman, A. (2012). Child–parent psychotherapy and traumatic exposure to violence. *Zero to Three, 32*, 20–25.

Schechter, D. S., & Willheim, E. (2009). Disturbances of attachment and parental psychopathology in early childhood. *Child and Adolescent Psychiatric Clinics of North America, 18*(3), 665–686.

Stern, D.N. (1995). *The motherhood constellation: A unified view of parent–infant psychotherapy*. New York: Basic Books.

Toth, S. L., Maughan, A., Manly, J. T., Spagnola, M., & Cicchetti, D. (2002). The relative efficacy of two interventions in altering maltreated preschool children's representational models: Implications for attachment theory. *Development and Psychopathology, 14*, 877–908.

Toth, S. L., Rogosch, F. A., Manly, J. T., & Cicchetti, D. (2006). The efficacy of toddler–parent psychotherapy to reorganize attachment in the young offspring of mothers with major depressive disorder: A randomized preventive trial. *Journal of Consulting and Clinical Psychology, 74*, 1006–1016.

Van der Kolk, B. A. (2005). Developmental trauma disorder. *Psychiatric Annals, 35*, 401–408.

Van Horn, P. & Lieberman, A.F. (2010). *Child–parent psychotherapy: A manual for trainers*. Unpublished manuscript.

Van Horn, P., Osofsky, J. D., Henderson, D., Korfmacher, J., Thomas, K., & Lieberman, A. F. (2012). Replication of child–parent psychotherapy in community settings: Models for training. *Zero to Three, 33*, 48–54.

Zero to Three. (2005). *Diagnostic classification of mental health and developmental disorders of infancy and early childhood: Revised edition (DC: 0–3R)*. Washington DC: Author.

7

CPP with an Infant Boy in the Child Welfare System

The Case of Claudia and John W.

Michele M. Many

with commentary by Patricia Van Horn and Alicia F. Lieberman

BACKGROUND INFORMATION

Child protective services (CPS) and the local dependency court referred Claudia W., a 21-year-old Hispanic female, and John W., her 10-month-old son, for child–parent psychotherapy (CPP). CPP was conducted in the context of John and Claudia's involvement in the child welfare system because of Claudia's failure to provide adequate care for John, who was medically fragile and diagnosed with failure to thrive. CPP was one the requirements for Claudia's reunification with her son.

By 10 months of age, John was exposed to several traumas and stressors including a lengthy stay in the neonatal intensive care unit (NICU), multiple illnesses and surgeries, and separation from his mother during his hospitalizations and subsequent removal from her care by CPS. John presented with serious developmental issues resulting from complications at birth and medical issues related to a shunt placed to address hydrocephaly (excessive fluid in the brain). Given John's medical complications, he required supervision and monitoring.

Neither John nor Claudia presented with any history of mental health treatment or diagnoses. Claudia's current symptoms included depression,

121

difficulties forming and maintaining peer and supportive relationships, poor-quality interactions with her children, and inappropriate developmental expectations of John. John demonstrated symptoms of developmental delays, emotional dysregulation (e.g., difficulty soothing even with the help of a care-giver), and symptoms of depression (e.g., flat affect and diminished pleasure in interactions and activities), especially when with his mother.

ASSESSMENT

Review of Records

Hospital Records Review

According to hospital records, John was born more than a month prema-turely, remained in the neonatal intensive care unit for more than a month after his birth, and had repeated subsequent hospitalizations. Claudia sel-dom visited John at the hospital except when mandated to attend trainings to learn how to tend to his medical needs. During these trainings, Claudia complained about feeling "imprisoned" and repeatedly asked when she could leave. During a particular month-long hospitalization, Claudia spent only two nights with John, and on these nights, staff noted that Claudia referred to John as "mean" and ignored him. Staff also reported that those family mem-bers whom Claudia identified as her primary support system never visited John while in the hospital.

CPS Records Review

When CPS initially received a report of medical neglect, it was noted that John had three hospitalizations over the course of 4 months. He was mark-edly underweight when admitted to the hospital, but gained weight while hospitalized and was subsequently diagnosed with nonorganic failure to thrive. Based on this initial CPS investigation, Claudia received support-ive services to aid in caring for her son. Records from home health services indicated that their providers eventually refused to offer in-home services, reporting that they felt unsafe due to hostility and repeated verbal threats by family members living with Claudia. Shortly thereafter, CPS received a report that John was left at home unsupervised. Upon investigation, CPS found John alone in the home, asleep, uncovered in his crib, and running a high fever. Inspection of his equipment and medications indicated that they had not been used and administered as directed. Claudia was later located at a neighbor's home. Both 6-month-old John and his 24-month-old sister Jade were placed in CPS custody and, because no placement with relatives could be found, CPS placed John and his sister in a dually certified foster home (certified for both foster care and adoptive placement). By the time John was referred for CPP, his sister, who did not have medical problems, was reunited and living with Claudia.

Observations and Information from Initial Meetings

During her initial interview, Claudia was pleasant and cooperative, although she displayed some initial mistrust of the clinician, which was understandable given that she was court referred for services. However, after her initial appointment, Claudia's demeanor became more relaxed, and she more readily shared information about her family and her life. While Claudia was a 21–year-old woman of average intelligence, her clothing, judgment, interactions with others, and manner were immature; she behaved as if she were in her early to mid-adolescence.

Ten-month-old John presented as happy and engaged when with his foster mother but was lethargic, anxious, and fretful when with his biological mother. Notably, when he was distressed and both Claudia and his foster mother were present, John preferentially interacted with his foster mother. When John attempted to obtain reassurance or comfort from Claudia, her responses were inconsistent.

Formal Assessment

The Working Model of the Child Interview (WMCI; Zeanah, Benoit, Barton, & Hirshberg, 1996) and the face-to-face–still-face (still-face) procedure (Tronick, Als, Adamson, Wise, & Brazelton, 1978) were used to assess the mother's and foster mother's relationships with John. The WMCI is a structured interview administered to caregivers that was designed to elicit caregivers' attributions regarding their children. The still-face paradigm allows observation of an infant's behavior and affective response during a series of interactions with a caregiver. The caregiver and child are first observed interacting while face-to-face; then the caregiver is asked to maintain a "still face" and not respond to the infant in any manner; finally, the caregiver is asked to resume interaction with the infant.

Behavioral Observation of John and Claudia

During the still-face procedure, Claudia smiled at John, talking to him in a high-pitched but cheerful tone of voice and telling him how much she missed him. John looked at Claudia for a moment and then smiled briefly. Claudia's attempts to interact with John were noted to be moderately intrusive; for example, she thrust her face toward him, abruptly, saying "Boo!" At times,

Claudia demonstrated moderate affective attunement by mirroring John's movements and vocalizations; at other times, however, Claudia did not seem to read John's cues. For example, John averted his gaze on several occasions, and Claudia responded in a teasing manner and chastised him for not looking at her. John exhibited distress by sucking on his fist for the remainder of the interaction portion of the assessment. The clinician interpreted this behavior as John's attempt to self-soothe in the presence of an overwhelming mother. When Claudia stilled her face, John exhibited mild confusion, then distress by kicking his feet. When Claudia resumed interacting with John, he continued to suck on his fist and looked around the room, periodically looking at Claudia, then averting his gaze again. To the clinician, this behavior indicated that he was unable to use his mother to help him soothe and regulate his affect when distressed. Claudia did not read John's cues accurately and continued to interact with him in an intrusive manner.

Behavioral Observation of John and His Foster Mother

It is important to note the contrast between the still-face procedure with John and his biological mother and the still-face procedure with John and his foster mother. During the exercise, John's foster mother smiled and sang hymns in a soft voice, swaying and making rhythmic hand movements. John smiled in return and followed his foster mother with his eyes, gazing at her face and then at her hands. As her face went still, John's expression registered confusion, then mild distress as he sucked on his fist and kicked his feet. When the foster mother resumed interacting with John by singing and talking soothingly, John smiled guardedly, then more fully. His distressed movements decreased; he relaxed, and his face brightened at the foster mother's singing. John waved his hands, and the foster mother mirrored this movement, indicating their resumed attunement with each other.

Interview with Claudia

In her WMCI, Claudia described John's birth and first days at home following his release from the hospital as "scary" and "difficult." She reported worrying that "something will happen to John," that "nobody will like him because of his condition," and that "he's coughing all the time and I don't know why . . . he'll throw up, and I'll be scared." Claudia strongly identified with John, which was of particular interest since she reported preferring her daughter Jade and referred to John as the "mean one." She reported that John physically resembled her, while her daughter resembled her brother. She predicted that, like her, John would be "the black sheep of the family" while Jade, like her brother, would be the favored child. Claudia expressed concern that her family members would expect John to take care of them as they had expected her to do. Similarly, she worried that people would take advantage of John, explaining that "they can mistake your kindness for weakness."

Claudia rejected the notion that John had any special needs or developmental delays. Interestingly, Claudia was able to accurately describe John's medical equipment and delineate his daily care requirements; however, she also asserted that there was nothing wrong with him. This demonstrated a good cognitive understanding along with an affective denial of John's special needs. Claudia's denial interfered with her ability to adequately care for her son or to recognize when his medical condition became life threatening. For example, her psychological rejection of his medical vulnerability caused her to ignore his need for close monitoring of his shunt and his vulnerability to running sudden high fevers. Ignoring John's medical issues by leaving him at home while she visited a neighbor nearly resulted in his death.

TREATMENT PLANNING

Treatment goals were discussed with CPS and with Claudia. The clinician recognized that because the treatment was court ordered, Claudia may have felt some pressure to agree with the goals of treatment despite the clinician's explanation that she had the right to decline part or all of the services offered. It was mutually agreed that treatment would be dyadic (with Claudia and John). Treatment would focus on increasing Claudia's capacity to appropriately read and respond to John's cues, improving her ability to ensure John's safety, and enhancing her sense of competence and agency as a parent. The clinician considered that developmental guidance would be an important modality to address safety concerns. For example, an early safety goal was to help Claudia develop and implement a realistic schedule of care to ensure that John's complex needs were met. To achieve this goal, the clinician would help Claudia understand and accept appropriate developmental expectations for John given his medical problems. Therapy would also need to address Claudia's own painful childhood experiences since they interfered with her ability to appropriately meet her son's physical and emotional needs and informed her working model of John as a "mean" child.

TREATMENT COURSE

CPP was conducted over a 3-year period. There was, however, a 6-month interruption in treatment due to the displacement of both Claudia's family and the foster family after a natural disaster affected the region. Further challenges arose for Claudia as she struggled to navigate the child welfare and judicial systems.

Building Trust

Claudia initially experienced difficulty in regularly attending her therapy appointments, giving reasons such as illness, oversleeping, and conflicting appointments. These episodes of resistance were explored in several individual therapy sessions during which Claudia was able to state that she resented the involvement of CPS in her life and wished that they would simply return John to her and leave her alone. Around this time, the clinician learned that Claudia had not experienced affective attunement with her own parents. While empathizing with Claudia's feeling (i.e., her frustration), the clinician reflected that Claudia would have an opportunity to feel affective attunement in treatment. This experience might, in turn, enable Claudia to provide that same attunement to her son. The clinician also modeled appropriate attention to the safety needs that resulted in John's placement in CPS custody. Together, the clinician and Claudia examined the reasons why CPS could not realistically return John to her custody without her completing the requirements set forth by the court. The clinician also encouraged Claudia to attempt a more balanced view of her predicament by recognizing that both she and CPS were contributing to the obstacles with which she struggled.

During the third individual session, Claudia appeared visibly depressed, as evidenced by her sloppy attire, disheveled appearance, poor eye contact, lethargic responses, and reported despair about not having her son in her care. The clinician provided emotional support and offered to link Claudia with psychiatric services to further assess the severity of her depression. Through these conversations Claudia slowly began to disclose more about the "ghosts in her nursery." She reported feelings of isolation and "differentness" within her family of origin as well as feeling like the least-favored child. Claudia's current issues with CPS revived these feelings of inadequacy, and she shared these feelings with the clinician, explaining that members of her family were upset with her because of her involvement with CPS. These disclosures increased the clinician's empathy for Claudia and facilitated the CPP goal of maintaining an empathic, supportive, and consistent therapeutic environment. The disclosures also highlighted the importance of considering a client's current behavior in the light of her past.

As therapy progressed, Claudia became less defensive and was able to explore her feelings about her painful childhood so that her current beliefs were less affected by these past experiences. For example, during one session, Claudia admitted that she did not trust her CPS worker because the worker was of a different nationality and also resembled Claudia's brother.

This insight allowed Claudia to see the CPS worker in a more positive light, and they were subsequently able to work more productively together. Through the work in these early sessions, Claudia also developed sufficient trust in the clinician's ability to not only tolerate but also sensitively respond to her emotional states and beliefs. This trust permitted Claudia to more fully disclose inner struggles that were interfering with her ability to cope with the stress of John's removal from her care and were triggering inappropriate and self-defeating responses to service providers.

During these early sessions, Claudia began to disclose details about the unsafe, unpredictable childhood that she had experienced with her own family of origin. She described lifelong verbal abuse and reflected that these "ghosts in the nursery" (Fraiberg, Adelson, & Shapiro, 1975) continued to affect her current interactions with her family. She also reported feeling ashamed for having given birth to a child with medical and developmental problems. Furthermore, on the rare occasion when Claudia did acknowledge John's disability, she expressed that she felt like she was being punished by having a sick child.

Beginning from Simplicity

After Claudia attended several individual therapy sessions, her symptoms of depression decreased and her relationship with her CPS worker began to improve. In the early dyadic CPP sessions, the clinician "began from simplicity," a CPP maxim. At first, the clinician simply observed the quality of interaction between Claudia and John, noting when Claudia responded appropriately to his cues. The clinician also noted that Claudia began to reliably intervene to ensure John's safety by either verbally or physically moving him away from unsafe activities. During the early dyadic sessions the clinician often used "speaking for baby" (Carter, Osofsky, & Hann, 1991), an intervention in which the clinician helps the caregiver recognize her child's needs and desires by verbalizing what the child might say if he had the capacity. For example, when Claudia held John in her lap and sang to him, the clinician said "Oh mama, I love it when you hold me and sing to me." This nondirective intervention allowed Claudia to develop empathy for John, to take John's perspective, and to see John as a unique individual who responded to her interactions with him. It also helped Claudia view John's behavior differently by allowing her to better understand the meaning of his nonverbal communication.

While Claudia began to show improvement in her ability to meet John's physical and emotional safety needs, on some occasions, she continued to struggle in this area. For example, during one session when John climbed onto an unstable chair, the clinician observed Claudia to see whether she would intervene. When Claudia failed to respond to the unsafe situation, the clinician took action, which both ensured John's safety and modeled appropriate behavior for Claudia. First, the clinician told John "feet on the floor" in order to ensure John's safety and to model this behavior for Claudia. When John did not respond, the clinician walked over, took his hand gently, and helped him get off the chair. When John sat in the chair, the clinician thanked him for doing so. Claudia observed this interaction and afterward was receptive to guidance about setting limits with John when he engaged in unsafe activities. In subsequent sessions, with guidance and encouragement from the clinician, Claudia supervised John more effectively while experimenting with setting limits when John engaged in unsafe activities.

It was noteworthy that Claudia did not use the words *Mom* or *Mama* when referencing herself while talking to John. This was particularly poignant since Claudia was deeply wounded and angered when John and his sister referred to the foster mother as "Mama." The clinician reflected on Claudia's choice to have her children call her by her first name and wondered aloud how the children would be able to identify her as their mother if they called her by her given name, especially in a household where there were other female caregivers of similar ages. Claudia balked at this idea, feeling that her children should "know" that she was their mother, but she also agreed it could be confusing for them and began to instruct them to call her "Mama." This intervention served the CPP goal of promoting safety within the caregiving relationship by clarifying child–caregiver roles. It also served to reinforce Claudia in her role as "Mama," a nurturing maternal figure, a role that had previously been usurped by older female relatives.

Strengthening the Relationship through Developing Reflective Capacity

Although Claudia previously regarded John as a "mean" child, her ability to perceive him as a unique individual with a need for love and care improved. She no longer perceived him simply as a replica of herself. Concurrently, Claudia's internal representation of John became more positive, and John seemed to internalize his mother's representation of him as "good." The dyad was observed to engage in more positive interactions, which furthered both mother's and child's needs for each other's positive regard. As a whole, their interactions changed from primarily disengaged to more pleasurable, with increased periods of reciprocity.

Claudia proved to be very curious and receptive to developmental guidance and learning about her children as individuals. For example, she began coming to each session with a story about something that had happened either to herself, a friend, or a relative and their child. She often asked questions, demonstrating her desire to better understand her own and other children's behaviors. For example, Claudia stated that she had put a friend's toddler in the back seat of a car with another small boy in preparation for a trip to a park. She described that her friend "played" with the children by hiding below the children's line of sight and popping up in their window to startle them. Claudia told the clinician that she did not understand why the children became so upset when this happened. Claudia's curiosity and questions created the opportunity for the clinician to provide developmental guidance about how children of different ages and temperaments may react differently to being startled. The clinician and Claudia discussed how an older child might giggle at being startled, but a young child is likely to be frightened, feel unsafe, and need reassurance from a known caregiver in order to recover. Claudia's face lit up with understanding. She responded, "So he won't be scary (easily frightened) when he gets older?" The clinician explained that with consistent emotional support, a child who experienced developmentally appropriate fear could develop confidence by using a caregiver as a secure base to reestablish a sense of safety, and resultantly master the fear. Claudia delighted in learning and took pride in sharing what she learned with others in her community. Each week she proudly told the clinician that she had taught a friend or cousin what she had learned in the previous session.

Claudia's active interest and participation in sessions as well as the support she received from the clinician enabled her to gain empathy for and to better attune to John when he was upset or frightened. She was also able to imagine what might frighten him despite his limited ability to verbalize. Furthermore, by teaching what she learned to others, Claudia demonstrated an increased sense of agency and mastery as a caregiver. This resolution was particularly encouraging given Claudia's prior inability to take either of her children's perspectives or shield them from frightening situations. For example, when the clinician made her initial home visit to Claudia's house, Claudia was sitting on the sofa with her daughter Jade, who was then 2 years old, watching a movie with graphic violence on a large-screen television. At this time, Claudia was not aware that the gory images and loud screams and noises were frightening Jade, even though the little girl sat very still and watched the screen with a flat affect. Seeing the improvement in Claudia's desire and ability to understand and meet her children's emotional needs was a significant accomplishment that was very rewarding to both Claudia and the clinician.

Addressing an Intractable Ghost

As the quality of Claudia's interactions with John improved, and she more fully took on the role of "Mama" to her son, Claudia's inability to accept John's disability was periodically revisited, and the clinician gently tested Claudia's openness to exploring this painful dilemma. Claudia was able to further explore her close identification with John through her experience of being the "black sheep" of her family. In an earlier session, Claudia reported that her siblings all closely resembled her father in both coloring and body type while she did not, and she was often teased and excluded because of this. The clinician questioned Claudia about this further, and Claudia acknowledged that she resembled her maternal grandmother in both coloring and body type. Although the clinician explained this phenomenon as common in many families, Claudia's sense of rejection by her siblings and parents was palpable. She viscerally felt that any acknowledgement of John as "different" would ensure that he would suffer as much, or possibly more, than she had when young. This particularly baneful "ghost" was clearly determined to cast its shadow on the next generation.

When the subject of John's shunt or his daily care was broached, Claudia continued to demonstrate the paradoxical ability to describe his medical condition and outline his daily care needs in detail, while also categorically asserting that there was nothing wrong with him and that he would be "normal" once the shunt was removed. This contradiction spoke to the blinding quality of her fear for John. The shunt removal surgery had long been planned, but was repeatedly delayed due to recurrent declines in John's health after visits with his mother, during which he did not receive adequate care. This was a salient issue because neither the court nor CPS was comfortable with returning John to Claudia's custody until she could care for him appropriately. Both systems believed that John's shunt presented the greatest risk of injury while under Claudia's care since constant monitoring of John's mental status, along with frequent visual inspections of the shunt, were required to ensure his safety. If this was not done regularly, he could die from infection. Once John had his surgery, however, his postsurgical needs would primarily be for therapies to address his developmental delays, which could be provided by home health services and later at school. Thus CPS and the court indicated that John might be safely returned to Claudia once his shunt was removed. However, the ongoing delays of this pivotal surgery prolonged John's ability to achieve stability in his placement, and he had at that point been in foster care for more than a year. The court considered limiting Claudia's visits in order to permit John time to stabilize for surgery; however, the court also decided that this would be overly punitive to Claudia and would violate her rights.

Treatment in Context: A Hurricane Strikes the Community

As plans were being made for John's surgery, a hurricane struck the area, prompting the evacuation of both Claudia's family and the foster family (John evacuated with his foster family). As a result of the prolonged disruption of infrastructure, basic and support services, and family systems, more than 6 months elapsed before the clinician reunited with Claudia and John. It would have been ill advised to resume therapy with Claudia without first allowing her to process and integrate her experience of this disaster. Therefore, the clinician met with Claudia individually to allow her to talk freely about her experience during her evacuation, displacement, and return to the city. In her first individual session after the hurricane, Claudia described a harrowing experience of a chaotic, last-minute evacuation before the storm. She reported being housed in shelters and with relatives until she and her family could return to their home. Notably, in telling this story, Claudia demonstrated the ability to understand how her daughter experienced the evacuation and return to the devastated city. She talked about the ways she worked to physically and emotionally protect Jade from potentially traumatic experiences, when possible, and integrate them when not.

During a session attended by Claudia, John, and Jade, Claudia continued to talk to the clinician about her evacuation experience. In order to encourage Claudia to jointly engage with her children during the session, the clinician brought the children into the conversation by listening to Claudia describe Jade's experience and then speaking directly to John and Jade. She reflected how scary the experience must have been for both of them and stated how glad she was that each child had an adult with them to keep them safe.

Given that the foster mother evacuated with John, the clinician felt it was important to have collateral sessions with John and his foster mother in addition to the sessions with John and Claudia. These sessions would help John make sense of this additional trauma with the support of both his biological and foster mothers. John's foster family also reported experiencing helplessness and fear as they stayed in a large hotel in the city during the hurricane and evacuated after the storm had passed. Based on John's responses after the storm and in the presence of his foster mother, the clinician judged that the foster mother provided John with a sense of safety during the storm. As a result, he did not exhibit any additional trauma symptoms.

Resuming Treatment: Focus on Areas of Strength and Areas of Concern

Following the hiatus forced by the hurricane, Claudia's treatment progress and goals of therapy were reassessed. Claudia had shown significant improvement in several areas of the original treatment goals. She was better able to appropriately and supportively respond to John's cues for attention and to set appropriate limits when he engaged in unsafe activities; she also displayed an increased sense of competence as a parent and had affirmed her role as "Mama" to her children. Her grasp of developmental norms was much improved, and she had gone further by taking the information gleaned in her therapy sessions to her friends and relatives. Becoming a teacher to them increased her sense of competence and agency within her community. Yet Claudia had not met a primary goal, one that would have a great impact on her ability to safely care for her son. Despite her knowledge of the instrumental medical care required because of his shunt, Claudia could not meet John's medical needs. For example, when John was hospitalized after the hurricane due to an allergic reaction to a medication, Claudia once again rarely visited John at the hospital. When the clinician asked about this, Claudia protested that she was at the hospital "all the time." The clinician went to the hospital and reviewed the nurse's notes, which documented who was at John's bedside on an hourly basis. Claudia was documented to have visited only one out of every 3 to 5 days, and only for brief visits of approximately an hour. This behavior indicated that being directly confronted with her son's fragile physical state overwhelmed Claudia and led to ongoing denial of his condition.

Focusing on the Past/Focusing on the Present

The clinician understood Claudia's inability to fully accept and respond to John's disabilities as related to her feeling rejected by her family. Through interactive discussion, exploration, and reflection, the clinician helped Claudia recognize the negative impact that her past was having on her relationship with her son. She helped Claudia differentiate the past from the present and herself from her child. The clinician also helped Claudia understand that, although John may have lifelong developmental delays, he need not relive her childhood pain. While addressing past issues, the clinician also supported Claudia in cultivating current relationships. For example, the clinician encouraged Claudia to improve her current familial relationships when possible and encouraged her to reach out to John's foster mother as a resource to help her improve her skills in meeting John's current care needs.

During the following sessions, the clinician used John's repeated illnesses and hospitalizations after his visits with Claudia as a port of entry to explore her ambivalence about his medical condition and developmental delays, especially through the lens of Claudia's own fears of being different, isolated, and rejected by her family. Claudia struggled with her fear of her family's reaction to John and with her sense that John's delays and medical issues were a "punishment" for her own "differences" within her family. The clinician empathized with the pain Claudia experienced and stated that it was not her fault that her family was so harsh with her. The clinician further reflected her own experience of Claudia as an intelligent, loving, and beautiful young woman who loved her child and was trying to do her best to care for him. Claudia was encouraged to explore the differences in John's experiences and her own, recognizing how John's experience was already different from hers and reflecting on John's having a mother who loved him and was protective of his feelings. This highlighted the difference between past (Claudia's) and present (John's) experiences.

The clinician noted that while the themes Claudia explored through the months of treatment were the same, over time Claudia gained a deeper understanding of her experiences, herself, and her children and was able to recognize the increasingly complex patterns of her own and her children's behaviors and relationships. With this insight, Claudia began to demonstrate in many ways her ability to assume a caregiving role for her children. For example, she identified the times she had intervened when she felt others treated John as "different" and described how her interventions helped John to be treated like the other children. The clinician explored how Claudia was creating a safer emotional environment for John than she had experienced as a child. With these reassurances, Claudia was able to further discuss her ambivalence about accepting the reality of John's medical condition, which contributed to the repeated delays of John's surgery. She was also able to verbalize that these delays, in turn, prolonged the possibility of John's returning to her care.

In order to provide Claudia with concrete support enabling her to visualize taking on the daily responsibilities associated with caring for John's medical and developmental needs, the clinician worked with the foster parent to develop a functional analysis of John's daily, weekly, and monthly care needs and medical appointments. This analysis was discussed with Claudia over the course of two sessions, and her reactions were processed. Once again, Claudia understood her son's schedule and was able to outline it with little effort. Claudia's compliance with his care during his visits improved slightly, but remained poor.

TREATMENT COMPLETION

At this point, John's physicians determined that his shunt should remain in place indefinitely. During the next court hearing, it was determined that Claudia's compliance with many aspects of her case plan were good, that her relationship with John had markedly improved, and that she had shown some improvement in her functional care of John. Furthermore, because John had physically grown and become stronger, he was determined to be less medically vulnerable. Given these considerations, CPS began to allow Claudia extended visits with John. The clinician worked with CPS and the dependency courts to advocate for a minimum of 3 months of close monitoring by CPS. However, the clinician also expressed her concerns about Claudia's ability to adequately care for John since she had a history of neglecting John's medical needs and had shown limited improvement in managing his daily care regimen. The goal of these visits was to provide the opportunity for Claudia to demonstrate that she could manage John's care over several days. The clinician communicated to Claudia the hope that she could rise to this challenge and encouraged Claudia to demonstrate to the court that she could take care of her child.

The extended visits were not without issues, but Claudia demonstrated increased openness to discussing problems as they arose. In addition, her level of cooperation with her CPS worker was much improved given her decreased defensiveness and increased feelings of confidence as a parent. Claudia sought the worker's and the clinician's guidance regarding decisions about supervision of the children, such as when she could leave them with others and with whom. In her dyadic (with John) and triadic (with John and Jade) therapy sessions, Claudia's progression toward feeling competent as a parent was demonstrated by her asking fewer questions and telling more stories about her exploits with John and Jade. She talked confidently about outings and birthday parties they had enjoyed, how she dealt with an issue at John's school, and how much her family loved John. Claudia's judgment remained variable, but it was promising that she was able to use CPS and the clinician as supports to help her navigate challenging situations.

Although Claudia's fears for John because of his disabilities remained a concern, they receded somewhat as a result of her family's reportedly warm affection for John. In some ways Claudia may have come to feel redeemed by John—her family loved him and accepted him without reservation. Thus Claudia may have felt that her past experience of rejection by family members was healed through their love of John, who was a part of her. The clinician reflected Claudia's successes and congratulated her on her progress.

As therapy progressed toward termination and the court moved toward reunification of John with his mother, the clinician explored the progress Claudia had made toward treatment goals. The clinician recognized the importance of mindfully moving toward termination, especially given Claudia's experience of loss related to her having suffered deep wounds from rejection by her family members. Therefore it was of utmost importance that termination of her therapy be handled with great sensitivity and forethought. With this in mind, the clinician discussed with Claudia how the end of treatment would involve losing the supportive relationship that they had developed. Furthermore, although completing and moving beyond her involvement with CPS and foster care was a triumph for Claudia, it would involve her letting go of a stable support system, including the CPS worker, who had remained constantly involved throughout Claudia's case plan, and

John's foster mother, who had in many ways mentored Claudia and been another consistent and stable presence for her. While Claudia minimized the emotional impact of these relationships, she did recognize that she would miss some aspects of them.

The clinician aided Claudia in taking John's perspective by reflecting on how these endings may affect him. Claudia was able to think about how the loss of these relationships would impact her son and said that she thought it would be hard for him. The clinician and Claudia discussed how to help John with these feelings; one way to help John transition from the nest of the foster home to the nest of his mother's home was to engage the foster parent as a mentor to Claudia. This was especially important given that John's foster mother had raised him from infancy. Together, the clinician and Claudia explored how John's foster mother had been a support not only to John but also to Claudia. The clinician asked whether Claudia thought she might want to maintain contact with the foster mother for ongoing support (something the foster mother had told the clinician she would like to do). Claudia agreed to think about this but acknowledged that she was not sure she was ready to make that decision.

By the end of treatment, Claudia had accepted the role of "Mama" to her son, and her depression decreased as her sense of parenting competency increased. As Claudia was more consistently able to accurately read and supportively respond to his needs, John's emotional and behavioral dysregulation decreased and his depression remitted. The course of this dyad's CPP treatment resulted in Claudia and John enjoying a much warmer and more mutually satisfying relationship with each other. Claudia gained more realistic developmental expectations of her children and was better able to meet their respective needs. While this application of CPP did not result in fully addressing and integrating the most salient issue with which Claudia presented (her own history of verbal abuse and being rejected as different by her family and her projection of this fear onto John), significant progress was made in this area. Through helping Claudia differentiate her experience from John's and through improved current relationships with her family, Claudia made sufficient progress in moderating her fears for John. With fewer fears about John's differences, Claudia was more able to accept them, allowing her to provide him with adequate care.

COMMENTARY

Few cases present greater complexities to a treating clinician than those involving children in foster care. Because CPP focuses on the child's relationship with his or her caregiver, it may be better suited than many modalities to resolving the conflicts in relationships made vulnerable by maltreatment or neglect and further compromised by separation. Children in foster care face an unresolvable existential dilemma. To whom should the child attach? Whom should she love, trust, and turn to for care and comfort? The younger the child, the more critical is his or her need to resolve this dilemma and form a caregiving relationship that supports the child's growing sense that the world is safe, that people are benign and responsive, and that the child is worthy of love and care. CPP can help children resolve this dilemma by providing a narrative to help them hold their biological parents in mind even as they are supported in learning to turn to a substitute caregiver who is there to meet their daily needs.

CPP clinicians working with children in foster care face a similar, if much less intense, dilemma. They must know which caregiving relationship they are to support. We recommend that clinicians form solid relationships with their child welfare agencies so that they can have candid conversations with child protection workers about the outcomes that workers forecast for children they refer for treatment. Two common patterns emerge. The first, the pattern exemplified by the case of Claudia and John, is that the clinician is asked to facilitate reunification of the child with his or her biological parent by working from the beginning to support and strengthen that relationship. The second pattern is that the clinician is asked to work initially with the child and his or her foster parent, stabilizing the placement. Then, as reunification approaches, the clinician is asked to transition the work and focus on the child and the biological parent to support the child's return home. Both of these clinical frames are clearly different from that on which CPP's evidence base was established. However either one can be used to deliver an intervention that is consistent with the fundamental principles of CPP.

This case study highlights the importance of utilizing the assessment period to deliberately establish a trauma frame for treatment. In the clinician's discussion of treatment planning, she stated that therapy should "when possible . . . address Claudia's own painful childhood experiences, which interfered with her ability to meet her son's medical and emotional needs. . . . " However, it was not clear that the clinician directly asked about the mother's trauma history during the assessment period. This primary assessment task would have been necessary in order to scaffold the mother's increasing understanding that adverse events in both her own and her child's life had a meaningful impact on their functioning. We believe that the child welfare setting may make it more emotionally challenging for clinicians to ask questions about the parents' lifetime trauma histories. Clinicians may fear that parents, who are mandated to treatment as a condition for reunification with their children, may view these questions as intrusive. It is not our experience, however, that this is necessarily the case. We have completed structural interviews eliciting lifetime experiences of trauma from dozens of biological parents seeking to reunite with their children as well as from the foster parents who were involved in the children's care. The child welfare context does not, of itself, preclude fidelity to this aspect of CPP. Rather, it argues for the use of reflective supervision, a core component of CPP, to work through any hesitance that clinicians might experience in directly addressing trauma so that a trauma frame to guide treatment can be established.

The clinician who treated Claudia and John adhered sensitively to many of the core domains and components of CPP. Foremost, she established an empathic relationship with Claudia, understanding that Claudia needed to experience herself as held and understood before she could open her heart to look past her own pain and frustration and truly understand John's dilemma. Second, she focused her work on translating John's cues and internal world for Claudia, supporting her in becoming more adept at understanding John and meeting his needs. Third, she worked collaboratively with Claudia, planning treatment goals with her and using interventions that engaged Claudia in a partnership focused on understanding John as well as her daughter.

The clinician adhered to the core CPP value of starting with simplicity, and this was a highly successful strategy in this case. Psychoeducation and developmental guidance helped Claudia gain a deeper and more flexible understanding of her children so that she became less dependent on the clinician's help to interpret their motivations and more confident in her own ability to take on this essential mothering role. The clinician was sensitive to the meaning of termination for someone who, like Claudia, had suffered many relationship losses in her lifetime and used the termination period to help Claudia begin to recognize the emotional weight that her relationships with the clinician, the foster mother, and the child protection worker held for her. Furthermore, during the termination period, the clinician guided Claudia in helping John manage his feelings about saying goodbye to these important people. In all of these critical ways, the treatment offered to Claudia and John was adherent to CPP and enabled Claudia to work through and overcome many of the internal conflicts that were standing in the way of her ability to care for John.

In spite of the successes reported in this treatment, we are left feeling concerned at its conclusion because of the reported "poor" quality of Claudia's compliance with John's medical care regimen during visits, even as the court determined that the visits should be extended and that John should go home to his mother. Our discomfort is not with the way that CPP was practiced in this case, but with what may be the "shadow" of CPP's focus on holding the parent–child relationship as the focus of intervention. In this case, John, a medically fragile child, had lived the first 3 years of his life with a foster parent to whom he appeared to be securely attached and who had provided him with excellent care. One wonders at a child welfare system that left him in foster care for so long, seemingly in contravention of legal mandates. Why did this system devote so much effort over so many years to restoring him to the custody of a biological mother who, although she had an intellectual understanding of the care he required, was consistently unable to provide it, putting him repeatedly at risk? We wonder whether there is something about CPP's focus on the relationship that makes it, particularly in child welfare cases, difficult for a clinician to advocate for the needs and safety of the child, even if it means losing the relationship that has been the focus of treatment.

Although the focus of CPP intervention is on the relationship, the clinician must be a steady advocate for safety within the relationship. Child welfare cases bring a complex set of players into the therapeutic field. Caregivers are subject to the demands of the child welfare agency and of the court. Child protection workers and judges come to the case with their own values about the importance of biological relationships and, often, with a hesitance to disrupt those relationships. Foster parents may be in a position in which they can also assert their feelings and wishes about what the child needs. CPP clinicians must balance the relationship that is the focus of their intervention, with all of these outside influences on that relationship. In the midst of that balancing act, they must keep an objective eye on the welfare of the child and on what is required for the child's safety and well-being. Meeting such a demand is not inconsistent with CPP's focus on the caregiving relationship. However, it does require the clinician, often with the active assistance of a reflective supervisor, to weigh the relationship she has worked so hard to develop and support against the child's need for safety. It may well be that the clinician in this case weighed those conflicting priorities, advocated on behalf of what she believed were the child's paramount needs, and chose not to write about that because she wanted to leave the emphasis of the chapter on the clinical work. If that is the case, it is our role as commentators to note the importance of this added element.

Review of the clinical work presented in this chapter convinces us that the modifications made to help children and caregivers manage the losses and transitions inherent to child welfare involvement do not, of themselves, diminish fidelity to CPP. Children and caregivers involved in the child welfare system can certainly be treated using CPP. The child welfare context does, however, demand that the clinician be vigilant lest the parent–child relationship be reified in its centrality and elevated over the safety of the child.

REFERENCES

Carter, S. L., Osofsky, J. D., & Hann, D. M. (1991). Speaking for the baby: A therapeutic intervention with adolescent mothers and their infants. *Infant Mental Health Journal*, *12*(4), 291–301.

Fraiberg, S., Adelson, E., & Shapiro, V. (1975). Ghosts in the nursery: A psychoanalytic approach to the problems of impaired infant-mother relationships. *Journal of the American Academy of Child Psychiatry, 14*(3), 387–421.

Tronick, E., Als, H., Adamson, L., Wise, S., & Brazelton, T. B. (1978). Infants' response to entrapment between contradictory messages in face-to-face interaction. *Journal of the American Academy of Child and Adolescent Psychiatry*, 17, 1–13.

Zeanah, C. H., Benoit, D., Barton, M. L., & Hirshberg, L. (1996). *Working Model of the Child Interview coding manual*. Unpublished manuscript.

8

CPP with a Preschool-Age Boy Living in a Residential Program for Women with Substance Use Disorders

The Case of Deanna and Brian C.

Amy R. Sommer and Eda Spielman

with commentary by Patricia Van Horn and Alicia F. Lieberman

BACKGROUND INFORMATION

Deanna C. and her two young children, Brian and Annie, were living at a residential program for pregnant and parenting women in substance use recovery when they were referred for child–parent psychotherapy (CPP). Brian had recently turned 4, and his younger sister Annie was 18 months old. They had just been reunified with their mother after spending 6 months in foster care. Deanna, age 28, was married to Charlie, age 29, the father of her children. He was living in a nearby sober house for men and visited the family one evening a week and on Sunday afternoons. The family was Caucasian and from a working-class community about 10 miles from the treatment program, so they were able to visit their home community periodically.

Approximately 1 month after Deanna began treatment at the residential program, the child services coordinator referred the family to CPP because of concerns about regressions in Brian's behavior. Deanna shared these concerns and described him as "clingy" since the reunification. Although the staff understood that time in foster care could cause some of Brian's difficulties, they were also concerned about Deanna's parenting. They described her as using fear as a primary form of discipline; for example, she told the children to stay close to her in the house for fear they might be "kidnapped." The staff also shared their impression that Deanna struggled with feelings of anger and frustration in the residential setting and wondered whether she might decline CPP.

When the clinician received the referral, she thought carefully with the staff about whom to include in the treatment. Although Deanna and Brian were the focus of the staff's concern, the clinician wanted to consider the possibility of including other family members. The residential staff thought Charlie would be an eager treatment participant, and his proximity and regular involvement with the children offered the opportunity to include Charlie in treatment and see the family in a variety of configurations. The clinician agreed with the staff that she would seek both Deanna's and Charlie's thoughts about whether to include Annie in their sessions. Leaving her out may have left more room to focus on Brian's presenting difficulties, but the clinician wondered whether Annie's stay in foster care at a critical time in the development of her attachment relationships may have affected her in ways the residential staff had not yet noticed.

TREATMENT SETTING AND INTERVENTION

A picture of the context for this family's treatment is helpful in understanding some of the challenges and opportunities related to CPP. The program where Deanna, Brian, and Annie were living housed a dozen families for an average stay of 6–8 months. Parents participated in a range of treatment services that supported their sobriety and prepared them to return to the community. Although the intention of the program was to focus on supporting residents in their parenting, the realities of staffing limitations and conflicting program goals meant that the needs of young children and the developing parent–child relationships were often lost to other priorities. Mothers came to the program with significant histories of trauma, mood disorders, and substance use. Most, like Deanna, had received only minimal treatment in the past and had few family or community supports.

Provision of CPP to program residents was made possible by grant funding awarded to a local agency, which provided technical assistance to the residential program, in partnership with an infant–parent treatment program where the clinician was employed and received supervision. The grant was designed to provide families with resources related to issues of trauma, attachment, and parenting within the context of recovery. Planning to provide CPP in a residential recovery program often felt daunting. Treatment length would be limited to 8 months at most, yet it would necessarily incorporate aspects of parents' extensive trauma histories and mental health needs.

The tandem realities of recovery and parenting presented a paradox: the desire to be a good parent was a primary motivation for seeking treatment and abstaining from drug use, but the stresses of day-to-day parenting were a significant challenge to maintaining sobriety. Early parenting in the context of recovery presented dual tasks of regulation. For example, newly in recovery, Deanna and Charlie needed to build their own capacities for coping with strong feelings while simultaneously managing the needs of two young children who could be easily dysregulated themselves. Along with the focus on emotion regulation, other CPP goals for this population included supporting the parent–child relationship in its capacities for safety, communication, and pleasurable interaction. Particular emphasis was given to facilitating parental reflective function—the capacity to understand intentions and motivations underlying behavior—as this is found to be a key intervention target for mothers in substance use recovery (Pajulo, Suchman, Kalland, & Mayes, 2006; Suchman, DeCoste, Leigh, & Borelli, 2010).

Working within a residential setting offered significant opportunities and challenges for the CPP project. At the residence where Deanna and her children lived, the focus on the clients' recovery process emphasized a culture of structured rules and consequences that was often at odds with the relational approach of CPP. The residential staff and CPP clinicians often had different understandings of the meaning of client's needs and behaviors. For example, program staff may have labeled a resident as manipulative and impose consequences, whereas the CPP clinician may have viewed the client as responding to a traumatic reminder and needing help in calming and expressing her feelings.

Children's needs could also be understood very differently. For example, when the residential staff referred Deanna's family to the CPP clinician, they asked that the clinician "talk with Deanna" about taking Annie's pacifier away, as they felt it was "babyish." In such instances, the clinician worked to understand the views of the residential staff while also using the important lenses of development, trauma, and attachment to help the staff understand the family's perspective. Regarding Annie's pacifier, the CPP clinician asked the residential staff to consider that it helped Annie meet needs related to separation, loss, and soothing.

Along with challenges in this residential setting, the milieu also offered some benefits, including its relative safety for the children and parents as well as ongoing supports for abstinence and recovery. The CPP work could unfold without some of the anxieties and uncertainties of treatment with this population in an outpatient setting. Deanna's clinician would know that Brian and Annie would be well cared for physically during their stay and that

Deanna would be attending groups to provide her with coping tools related to her addictions.

FAMILY ASSESSMENT

In the first of four sessions focused on intake, assessment, and treatment planning, the clinician met with Deanna and Charlie while the children were at daycare. The clinician explained that she was seeing families at the residential program who had expressed concerns about their children to the child services coordinator and mentioned Deanna's concern that Brian had regressed in his behavior. Charlie was immediately more talkative than Deanna. However, both parents actively participated in the session, stating that they worried that their son's behavior may be associated with his traumatic experiences. The clinician gathered a family history as well as a developmental history focusing primarily on Brian but also including Annie's experiences since the parents and clinician had decided that Annie should be a part of the treatment. The clinician considered how attachment relationships, development, and traumatic experiences colored the history and observations of the family (Lieberman & Van Horn, 2008). Importantly, she worked to maintain a sense of curiosity about behaviors, motivations, and feelings, so that she could remain open to "not knowing" and the opportunities for mentalizing—for considering the internal life of self and others—that this might offer.

As she heard Charlie and Deanna recount their children's history, the clinician reflected, "By sharing so much about Brian's past, you're helping the three of us begin to wonder together about his experiences in the present, what things might be like for him now." This kind of statement can also lessen parental shame as parents share past events that may be painful to face in the present. The second and third sessions involved meetings with each parent separately to discuss their own histories. Again, the clinician used a curious stance to facilitate the sharing of difficult history and traumatic past events. "I ask parents about their own past, as children who were cared for, so that we can think together about possible connections between those memories and your experiences now as a parent."

Finally, the family met with the clinician for a play session that included each child in a triadic play procedure similar to that used by Fivaz-Depeursinge and colleagues (Fivaz-Depeursinge, Corboz-Warnery, & Keren, 2004). In this paradigm, each parent spent 5 minutes playing alone with each child while the other parent turned his or her attention elsewhere. This allowed the clinician to observe the child's use of each of their parents and the dynamics of the four parent-child dyads contained in this family.

Background Information

Family History

After being in a relationship for 3 years, Deanna and Charlie married when they discovered they were pregnant with Brian. Deanna characterized the pregnancy as very much wanted, a way of filling the "empty feeling" she was experiencing following some conflict with Charlie and the recent death of her favorite cousin. Before becoming pregnant, she developed a dependency on alcohol and nonprescription stimulants but stopped using both of these around 6–8 weeks' gestation. She described an easy, uncomplicated pregnancy during which she attended regular prenatal appointments. However, at the time of Brian's birth, the strains in the family system were clear. On the night Brian was born, Charlie and Deanna's mother were high, and a neighbor had to take Deanna to the hospital. Deanna's sense of abandonment by Charlie would pervade the family's early life. She tried to parent effectively while Charlie was actively using substances, but was overwhelmed and relapsed to alcohol and then cocaine when Brian was approximately 4 months old.

Brian's early months were marked by chaos and the disappearance, metaphorically and in reality, of each of his parents. Deanna and Charlie used substances heavily, acknowledging in retrospect that they were difficult to rouse, lost consciousness, and were physically ill between highs. They moved seven times in Brian's first 2 years, and Charlie completed several multiday medical detoxification programs, leaving Deanna to care for Brian alone. When Brian was 2, the couple realized they were pregnant with Annie, and again Deanna stopped using, while Charlie alternated between street life and detoxification centers. Unlike their pregnancy with Brian, this one was not planned, and Deanna was hospitalized for dehydration and a severe flu. Annie was born early and with immature lungs, requiring an 8-day stay in the neonatal intensive care unit. Deanna and Charlie viewed Annie as a fragile baby who faced multiple mild illnesses in her short life. With the stresses of a toddler and a newborn at home, the family again fell into patterns of heavy substance use and crisis. Charlie was arrested for attempting to sell illicit substances and served a 9-month prison term. Child protective services became involved at this time, placing the children in foster care when Brian was 3½ and Annie was just 1 year old.

Parents' History

Brian and Annie would clearly be marked by their own traumatic experiences, but the clinician learned also of Charlie and Deanna's "ghosts" as they shared their own trauma histories (Fraiberg, Adelson, & Shapiro, 1975).

Deanna's History. Deanna's father abandoned the family when she was 3. Her mother was dependent on benzodiazepines for much of her childhood and had a series of different boyfriends, one of whom molested Deanna when she was 12. When Deanna told her mother about the abuse, her mother supported the legal prosecution but continued to visit her boyfriend in jail, leaving Deanna feeling both violated and unprotected. Deanna witnessed violence between her mother and most of her mother's partners.

Although the residential staff had described Deanna as angry and difficult to relate to, a sense of a more multidimensional mother who seemed hungry for support took shape during the intake process. As she noted Deanna's strengths and openness to being vulnerable in the therapeutic relationship, the clinician wondered which relationships from Deanna's past had contributed to this fuller picture. Consistent with the Angels in the Nursery Interview (Lieberman, Padrón, Van Horn, & Harris, 2005), the clinician explored: "We've talked about some times in your childhood that were very painful, and those events may come up again as we work together, but there also may be memories from your childhood that connect to positive experiences you would like to share with your children. Many parents can remember a time when they have felt especially close or connected to a grown-up, maybe a parent or maybe someone else close to them. I'm wondering if any memories come to mind for you that you could share, and that we might use together as move forward in our work?" Deanna responded by talking about a maternal grandmother who was a source of support and positive parenting for the children in the family.

A prior clinician may also have been an "angel." Deanna reported receiving "a few sessions" of counseling when her mother found out that she had been sexually abused. Deanna stated that these were helpful because she felt "someone listened to me." She described experiencing symptoms of depression, irritability, and hostility throughout her adolescence; she received a diagnosis of bipolar disorder when she was participating in an outpatient addiction treatment group. Deanna began taking an antidepressant and a mood stabilizer when she entered residential treatment.

Charlie's History. During intake, Charlie described his family of origin as "very normal" but later acknowledged a number of traumatic experiences in his family life. His father, who died when Charlie was 22, was an alcoholic who used extensive corporal punishment. Charlie reported having to come to terms at that point with the fact that his father had been physically abusive to his mother throughout Charlie's life. Charlie's two younger siblings both struggled with addiction, and one brother spent most of his teen and young adult years incarcerated. Charlie denied a history of mental health treatment, diagnosis, or pharmacotherapy. Both Charlie and Deanna had lost friends to heroin overdoses in recent years.

Parents' Perceptions of Trauma. When asked to reflect on how trauma had affected their lives, both parents identified their recent separation from their children as devastating. When they were removed, the children were placed together for 6 weeks in one foster home and 4 months in a second home. Charlie and Deanna did not know why they were moved. The parents seemed genuinely pleased that their children seemed to have been safe in foster care, saying to Brian and Annie, "they took good care of you." In discussion during supervision, however, the clinician was able to explore a more complex view of the family's separation, Brian and Annie's foster care experience, and the potential meanings for Charlie and Deanna. The clinician and supervisor formulated the question: Could the parents' assurances to their children serve a secondary defensive and protective function in avoiding any understandable, but hard to acknowledge, guilt they felt about their own responsibility for the removal?

Parent–Child Observations

During the fourth meeting, the family came together so that the clinician could attend to the strengths, abilities, and vulnerabilities of each family member in dyadic and triadic configurations. Assessment with four family members in the room can be complex, especially as each person's development, trauma history, attachment needs, and relational patterns must be considered. Still, the rich observations that can be gleaned more than compensate for the challenges.

Observation of Brian

Brian presented as bright and friendly, although overly affectionate with the clinician when he met her for the first time. He wanted to hug her goodbye and shouted "I'll miss you!" as he left the session. This reaction is common in children who have had multiple caregivers and can provoke inappropriate reciprocal responses from professionals who want to be affectionate in return. Brian had some difficulty maintaining attention, talking rapidly as he jumped from topic to topic and ignoring questions or redirections. However, he responded well to limit setting, particularly when supported by his father. He engaged easily in pretend play with a great deal of elaboration but had some difficulty maintaining a coherent theme. He was observed to play well with his sister with some support in resolving typical sibling difficulties. Brian's verbal, motor, and cognitive skills seemed adequate for his age.

Observation of Annie

Annie was just learning to walk and was very interested in exploring her environment. She was generally quiet but cried without distinct syllables when she was frustrated. She did not connect with the clinician for most of the session and seemed to avoid most connection with her parents. For example, she moved away from them when they approached her during free play and exerted control during collaborative tasks such as building a block tower. She did not seek proximity to either parent when she became upset by an interaction with her brother, and both parents seemed at a loss as to whether to comfort her.

Observation of Family and Dyadic Relationships

Deanna and Charlie had clear strengths that were observed during these assessment sessions. Despite the staff's concern that Deanna would avoid treatment, both she and Charlie took their commitment to attending treatment seriously. They worked together and approached many parenting tasks with thought and effort. They had established daily routines for their children and explained transitions and consequences carefully. However, both parents also faced challenges in responding to their children's needs. They seemed to minimize distress in their children, insisting that they stop crying when upset and using phrases like "you'll be fine" when the children were having difficulty. While Charlie was fairly permissive when setting limits, he called both children "crybaby" on several occasions. Deanna had extremely high, developmentally inappropriate expectations of Brian and frequently criticized or corrected him. In contrast to her expectations of Brian, Deanna referred to Annie as "my baby" and seemed to expect "babyish" behavior from her.

Deanna was also observed to have an intrusive style in play and sought to control many play themes. Even with the most unstructured of play, including blowing bubbles or playing with blocks, she was demanding and showed little joy. During the observation session, Deanna chose to use physical contact with each child only when disciplining or "play fighting." For example, her only closeness with Annie occurred when she pulled her over and took hold of her face, saying "I want you to look at me when I'm talking." Charlie's parenting style was relatively more relaxed; he seemed able to share times of pleasure with his children and to follow the pacing of their play. However, he acknowledged his uncertainty about his children's development since he had been absent for much of their young lives.

FORMULATION AND TREATMENT PLANNING

The assessment sessions provided a framework for beginning CPP with Deanna, Brian, and their family. With their background of trauma and substance use, Deanna and Charlie faced many challenges as parents. Life with their children had evolved into a pattern, familiar from their own pasts, of unpredictability, loss, and harm. Brian and Annie were resilient, but their development was faltering as the impact of chronic stressors, significant traumatic experiences, and strained relationships with their caregivers threatened to overwhelm their capacities for growth. The opportunity for CPP came at a time of reunification and hopefulness albeit in the context of ongoing fragility and stress.

As the clinician began to formulate the work for this family and bring her thoughts and questions to supervision, she kept in mind that Deanna and her children had faced many life experiences apart from each other and that both parents were reconnecting with their children after a significant and traumatic separation. At the same time, both children were making sense of parents who, now sober, probably seemed quite different from the parents they had come to know, however briefly, in their earlier time together. As the parents acknowledged an interest in "knowing" about their children and wanted information and support about what to expect when children reunify and regress behaviorally, the clinician thought that developmental guidance would be helpful early in treatment and could be delivered in a manner that that would not arouse parental defensiveness (Lieberman & Van Horn, 2005). When faced with difficult moments either in the treatment room or as described by the parents, the clinician planned to inquire, "What do you make of it when children do that?" With questions such as this, she hoped to foster a reflective and curious, rather than didactic, approach to understanding the children's development.

CPP sessions offered the possibility of an emotionally safe therapeutic space where family members could begin to find their way at this new point in their family life. To achieve this, the clinician created an atmosphere that could contain difficult feelings and facilitate the possibilities for pleasure in relationships. The clinician's relationship with Deanna would support Deanna's capacities for building trust, curiosity, and regulation that would be crucial tools in parenting Brian and Annie, as well as in maintaining sobriety. Through play, the children and parents would be helped to show their feelings and needs and be supported in building safe and mutually rewarding forms of relating.

Emotion regulation was conceived as a primary focus of the treatment. Deanna had spent many years using substances to manage her affect, and the use of these substances may have altered her brain chemistry in such a way that made regulation more difficult (Borelli, West, DeCoste, & Suchman, 2012). Managing strong feelings without substances was a major task confronting Deanna, made more difficult by the dysregulation she experienced when meeting the needs of her two young children. Her dysregulation was, in turn, hard on the children. The clinician wondered how emotionally difficult material, that would necessarily be raised during child–parent work, could become a trigger for relapse for one or both parents.

Exploring the session material in supervision helped the clinician track the parents' responses to particular questions or statements. Supervision also heightened the clinician's sensitivity to moments in the treatment where affect might be unspoken, hidden, or opaque to parents, the clinician, or both. Experiencing intense emotion outside of a chemical "high" is something that many people with substance use disorders find difficult; however, the work of parenting necessarily involves strong affect. The clinician felt that it would be beneficial to help Deanna and Charlie understand that improvements in their relationships with their children and increased confidence in their sobriety would mutually enhance each other. Parent–child treatment was expected to directly benefit their sobriety, and sobriety would, of course, be essential to improving their relationships with their children. Given Deanna's difficult relationship history, the clinician anticipated a long engagement period; however, she was also aware of Deanna's strengths. Deanna's warmth and openness with the clinician were positive predictors of her ability to quickly make use of the clinician as a coregulator in high-affect interactions with her children.

Deanna expressed little pleasure or enjoyment when her children sought independence and engaged in creative or exploratory activities. These difficulties were considered amenable to dyadic treatment. Play sessions were seen as a way to increase positive affect, and the clinician spent a great deal of time in early sessions "simply" facilitating age-appropriate play between family members, hoping to expand the ways in which Deanna could find joy in interactions with her children. From the beginning, the clinician spoke for both children and parents when they found pleasure, for example, exclaiming, "You laugh so hard when mom plays peek-a-boo with you!" or observing, "Your face lights up when Annie brings you a ball to throw."

The theme of disappointment in Deanna's relational world was another critical piece to consider in case conceptualization and treatment. Deanna identified many people who had disappointed her and was sensitive to feeling that her children did not want to play with her. She seemed both hurt by and connected to others through this feeling. This dynamic was seen in parallel with the treatment staff at the residence who expected her to disappoint the clinician by not attending treatment.

TREATMENT COURSE

Deanna and her family were seen for 28 sessions of CPP over the 8 months of their stay in the residential recovery program. As with any treatment over many months with a four-member family, the complex work involved different constellations and "story lines." Given the limitations of space, the focus here is on the major themes and relationships as the treatment evolved. Specifically, the focus of this case study is on Deanna and her relationships with her children and the CPP clinician. Other familial relationships (e.g., Charlie as a father and husband, as well as sibling interactions) are necessarily in the background. Because both staff and parents identified Brian as the child about whom they had the most concerns, attention to Annie in this case study is less prominent.

Developing a Shared Frame for Working Together

Being mindful of the many challenges this family faced, the clinician began with the most straightforward strategies for creating safety; she developed a therapeutic frame in which there was predictability in time and place as well as a child-friendly space to help the family feel safe and protected when they came to do the difficult work before them. Consistency in time, place, and frame felt particularly important in this case, as the family had moved many times and the children's serial separations and placements meant that every aspect of their daily lives had changed multiple times in only a few months. In addition, the family continued to encounter daily life experiences that hampered their ability to establish consistency, predictability, and emotional safety. Charlie was unable to attend the third session when he was asked to report for a urine toxicology screen. Similarly, the fifth session had to end early because of an unexpected requirement imposed by residential staff. These events felt beyond the family's control and caused the parents understandable frustration, anxiety, and anger.

When the consistency of the therapeutic frame was interrupted, the clinician was able to observe Deanna's response and better understand her relationship needs and dynamics. For example, during a snowstorm that occurred 2 months into treatment, the clinician was thoughtful about arriving to her appointment with Deanna on time, given the clinician's belief in the importance of therapeutic consistency for a mother whose experience of relationships had been unpredictable. Upon arrival, however, the clinician found that the family was ensconced in their room, not expecting the session to take place. When Deanna was called to the office, she presented a telling mix of surprise, gratitude, and defensiveness, saying sarcastically, "It's a *snow* day! *You're* not supposed to be here *today*!" The clinician responded with a warm greeting and acknowledged Deanna's surprise, noting to herself Deanna's difficulties with the unexpected and her pattern of expressing relationship connection in a defensive way. Deanna softened a bit and said that she thought it *might* be helpful to play. Her tone was grudging and, without understanding Deanna's experiences of disappointment over the course of her life, it might have been easy for the clinician to "take the bait" and retreat to an afternoon of paperwork and returning phone calls.

On another occasion, the clinician was forced to cancel a session because of her own illness. Toward the end of the next meeting, Deanna expressed her feelings about this, saying, "Of course, you'd pick last week to be out. Our kids are being *terrible*, and when you weren't here, they *acted up!*" At difficult moments like this, the clinician recalled previous discussions in supervision and responded by apologizing for the missed appointment and acknowledging Deanna's feelings as she said, "I'm disappointed also that I wasn't able to be here last week, and I hear your frustrations. Thank you for making it here today, even though it sounds like it's been a tough week. Sometimes, those are the weeks you and I, talking together, can learn the most from."

The clinician used a later supervision to explore her mix of feelings: guilt that she had let the family down, frustration that her efforts to be consistent did not seem appreciated, and anxiety that the family might find treatment inadequate and withdraw. Upon reflection, the clinician recognized that Deanna seemed to feel that the CPP work and the relationship with the clinician were both meaningful and helpful; however, Deanna maintained a stance of guardedness in her expression of need or dependence. The clinician understood this defensiveness as connected to Deanna's past experiences of hurt and abandonment in relationships and was open to seeing how their therapeutic connection continued to unfold.

Engagement through Play

This early treatment phase focused on helping the family feel comfortable being and playing together. Deanna and her family had very little experience in therapeutic treatment and had no experience with therapy involving the use of play. Given the unfamiliarity and the potential associations with being observed during child protective services visitations, the clinician wondered aloud about potential feelings of awkwardness and offered hope these would fade as trust was built. Phrases beginning "Some families have told me it can feel strange . . . " and ending with an invitation to hear

Deanna's experience, served to normalize feelings of discomfort and create an atmosphere where feelings could be discussed. The clinician also highlighted the value of using play to help the children reconnect with their parents after a separation and to help all the family members express feelings and thoughts about what had happened with their family. When introducing CPP, the clinician told the family that play would be "the work" and that "children can show us so much of what they know, and what they are concerned about, when we play with them." This explanation helped the family understand that "talk therapy" would not be the primary mode of intervention. Play in these early sessions was useful to observe and to wonder about, silently and sometimes aloud, the activities that each child and parent enjoyed as well as activities that were associated with more negative emotions and ways of relating.

During the family's early play sessions, the clinician learned about the children's ways of playing and being with their parents. Toddler Annie's more straightforward, physical play seemed enjoyable for both parents. Annie easily initiated interaction with her parents, and they quickly responded to her with pleasurable "wrestling" and rough-and-tumble play. When Annie disengaged from this kind of play, both parents had difficulty following her to a new activity. This left Annie playing on her own while either or both parents engaged more actively with Brian and his play.

Brian's early play was usually developmentally appropriate and brought him great joy; he would select an activity and explain his ideas to his parent (e.g., "Let's build a house with the blocks!") and could concentrate on the activity for a time. At times, however, he seemed overly compliant, particularly with his mother. For example, he followed her precise instructions with the blocks even when he struggled with fine motor control.

Fun and Fear

As the children and parents became comfortable in the play space, Brian's play began to elaborate, and he identified favorite toys: family dolls, dollhouse furniture, and small plastic animals. Brian was happy to narrate his play and involved his parents warmly, usually inviting an available parent to join him and offering them a role in play. When Brian invited the clinician to take a role, she encouraged a parent to join or gave her role to the parent, saying, "Maybe Mommy can be the mom, so I can help you both play."

When Brian's parents demonstrated that they could pretend with him, the clinician attended to issues of understanding, connection, and trust among the family members. It became clear that Deanna struggled to maintain a reflective stance while playing, becoming caught up in the play as if it were real; this impeded her ability to observe the play from a truly "pretend" place. In a few early sessions, for example, both children found that they could engage their mother in warm, silly play by making food for her in the pretend kitchen. They would carefully and elaborately take the play food from the refrigerator and offer it to her. Sometimes, she was able to be warm and silly in return, thanking them for the food and pretending to eat it with gusto, remarking on how much she enjoyed it. At other times, however, she would criticize the children's food choices and manners, saying, "That's not healthy!" or "Say 'please' first."

These moments presented challenges to the clinician as she watched two very young siblings struggle with their mother's harsh responses and unpredictable mood. By discussing these emotionally difficult situations with her supervisor, the clinician was able to reflect first during supervision and later with Deanna on the meanings of Deanna's harsh behavior. Building on the trust established in the first months and the exploration in supervision, the clinician was able to consider, in a fairly direct way, what it was like for Deanna at those moments. What was Deanna feeling when she shifted from play to stern "reality"? Why was it so hard for her to stay with these pretend themes? Gentle inquiries such as, "I noticed a big change in your tone just then . . . do you have a sense of what was going on inside you when that happened?" were used to help Deanna focus inward. Naming and making sense of the thoughts and feelings behind her harsh and controlling behavior supported Deanna's growing reflective capacity, which would later help her understand her impact on her children.

In talking about the "food play," Deanna was able to use the clinician's guiding questions to connect strong feelings about the children's actual food consumption during the day with her reactions in session. Deanna reported that both children were drawn to eating the snacks that she kept hidden in their single room; she labeled this as "sneaky" and "lying" and found it very upsetting. Using developmental guidance, the clinician offered support and thoughts around appropriate limit setting and ways to structure snack times. With a few simple adjustments to practical issues such as where the food was kept and what the children could have after they returned from daycare, Deanna's thinking shifted from seeing her children as sneaky and lying to thinking of them as curious and needing routine along with choices. On a deeper level, these conversations led to a discussion about Deanna's fears that she needed to control nearly everything in her children's lives so that they would be safe. Understanding these needs and fears and how they affected Deanna's ability to play with her children became an important focus of the CPP work. At the same time, the clinician, along with her supervisor, wondered about the possible links between Deanna's history of drug use and the emotional charge of fantasy play. How might her experience of her children seeking forbidden snacks relate to her own patterns of craving and addiction?

Might allowing immersion in fantasy be too evocative of the loss of reality in drug highs?

As treatment progressed, Brian began using play sessions to explore his feelings of fear and safety. At the beginning of one session when his father was absent and his mother was giving a snack to Annie, Brian chose to play with a family of plastic giraffes and blocks he arranged on the table. He invited the clinician to play the mommy giraffe and led a repeated game of hide-and-seek in which his baby giraffe would hide behind blocks so the mommy could find him. When Deanna was available to join, the clinician asked Deanna to be the mommy giraffe. Deanna and Brian agreed, and the clinician observed the play. Brian began the hide-and-seek game again, but Deanna immediately stopped the play and told Brian that she did not like it when he hid because she worried about him and did not know where he was. The clinician chose not to intervene, but to wait and see how the family would negotiate this situation. Brian whined that the animals were "just playing hide-and-seek" and beseeched his mom to play. She replied that she felt he was hiding because he did not want to play. The clinician commented, "Brian, you told us how much you wanted to keep on playing, and Mommy, you told us that you weren't so sure about this hiding play. It can be fun to pretend with the animals, but sometimes it reminds us of hard things." This seemed to help the dyad resume play.

As the game continued, Brian stacked some blocks and had the baby giraffe hide "way up high." Deanna attempted to stay with the play, asking "baby giraffe" to come down and be safe. Mother and son attempted to negotiate before Deanna seemed overwhelmed and again stopped the play, angrily telling Brian that he was not safe and she did not want to play with him if he was not going to listen and "play safely." She turned to the clinician and shared her frustration that "the kids don't listen."

It was apparent that Deanna saw the play not as Brian's effort to master issues associated with safety and protection but as a challenge to her authority as a parent and as a direct wish to put himself in harm's way. The clinician was aware that Deanna's difficulties with these themes were interfering with her capacity to engage in play with her son or to see her son's experience as separate from hers, and wondered about the multiple sources and meanings involved. At this difficult moment, the clinician began by being curious about Deanna's experience. Deanna struggled, barely able to manage her affect as she responded with pressured, angry speech about her children's wish to constantly do dangerous things, and the burden she felt as the only person who could protect them. As Deanna became tearful, the clinician gently pointed out how both Deanna and Brian had successfully managed a difficult moment and expressed confidence they would continue to do so. The clinician then arranged a time to meet with Deanna alone.

Deanna was able to use the individual session to consider the connections between her past experiences and present situation. As a young child, Deanna was both directly hurt and indirectly unprotected. Similarly, as a parent, Deanna's children had been in real danger, and she was not able to protect them. The clinician helped Deanna connect these past experiences to her present, in which feelings related to danger and loss of control at times overwhelmed her, leading to anxious and harsh responses. Deanna experienced her children's separation from her as a significant trauma, although she was not ready to acknowledge her part in their removal. During supervision, the clinician wondered whether the intensity of Deanna's sensitivity to issues of safety stemmed in part from her "knowing" on an unspoken level that she previously failed in this parental responsibility.

Over the next few months, as Brian's play grew to include increasingly "scary" themes, the clinician helped Deanna tolerate the play so that she could engage with her son and take a reflective rather than reactive stance. There seemed to be a strong link, which Deanna identified with help, between tolerating the unexpected in play, and Deanna's own experiences of loss of control and victimization. She identified her need to "know what was going to happen next" because of the many times that horrific events had been inflicted on her with unpredictability in both her childhood as well as her more recent past. When the family presented for treatment, Deanna acknowledged a great deal of worry about whether her children were safe living with strangers in a residential setting. These fears were likely fueled by the awareness that the children had been unsafe when in her care. She had resorted to controlling discipline and restrictive daily routines in an attempt to control her own anxiety. Learning to tolerate the unexpected in play had a paradoxical effect, and Deanna was able to be increasingly predictable with her children, offering them a more consistent emotional response. The focus on helping Deanna understand the sources of her fear and need for tight control helped her find ways to regulate her own feeling states.

Slow and Steady

Although there were times during the middle phase of treatment when the clinician wished that deeper connections between Deanna's past trauma and present parenting dilemmas could be addressed more quickly, the treatment continued to slowly progress. The clinician reflected with the family on their growing steps in treatment. She used the family's beginning challenges and needs as a point of reference, holding in mind all that the family members had to face each week just to tolerate coming together in one room for therapy sessions that focused on feelings and relationships. Brian's play around families and safety could be explored more openly, and both parents were developing new capacities to consider their children's experiences and feelings.

Annie was also developing many new skills. Early in treatment Annie was avoidant in relationships; however, at this point in treatment she actively elicited companionship in play, approaching her brother, mother, father, or the clinician with a smile and a verbal invitation for them to join a favorite activity. Her expressive language skills were noticeably improved, and both parents felt that she was better able to tolerate frustration and limit-setting in their day-to-day lives. One key to Annie's improved functioning could be seen in her relationship with her mother. During one session, when Annie wanted to play with bubbles, Deanna initially protested that they would be too messy. After some negotiation with the clinician regarding limits and rules, Deanna agreed to Annie's request. In an early treatment session, Deanna had used bubbles with her children, but the time was colored by her worries about mess and turn-taking, and there was no pleasure for any of them. During this later session, however, Deanna and Annie quickly found a rhythm with the bubbles that was truly playful for both of them. Deanna convinced Annie to let her blow the bubbles and encouraged Annie to catch and pop the bubbles, which she did joyously. The two came close together, in mutual enjoyment, as Annie grinned at her mother, anticipating the next blow of bubbles, and Deanna knelt on the floor, comfortable with getting down on her child's level and allowing the bubbles to pop all around her. With a warm smile, the clinician commented on their obvious joy, the ways that they mirrored each other's faces and lively gestures, and the connection they were obviously feeling with each other.

A Narrative for Moving On

After 7 months of treatment, Deanna and Charlie arrived for a session with the news that within the next week they hoped to move to another state where Charlie's extended family lived. Hearing of this plan, the clinician felt surprised by the sudden announcement and skeptical that the family's tenuous stability could survive such a move. The clinician wondered to herself, and later aloud in supervision, about possible links with patterns of impulsive and self-destructive behavior in the past. The shift from impulsivity to reflection and the development of regulatory skills were essential components of Deanna and Charlie's addiction recovery and were addressed in treatment. Following the parents' announcement, the next two sessions focused on slowing the action planning and encouraging Deanna and Charlie to reflect about their thoughts and feelings regarding this plan. Having a relationship context that enabled them to delay action and consider their thoughts, feelings, and decisions was a new experience for this couple who had made nearly every prior family decision in the face of chaos, powerlessness, and urgency. Could this be an opportunity to think about a choice, understand their own ideas and needs, and make meaning of their unfolding plans?

Their plans to move changed, however, when soon thereafter, a housing program in a nearby community announced an opening for a two-bedroom apartment, and the family was accepted immediately. The clinician used the next weeks to work together with the family on transition and termination since the grant requirements would not allow ongoing CPP services after they left the residential program. The parents told their children right away, as they were overjoyed by the news. Brian's play predictably and quickly turned to themes of home and moving; he used animals and people to show his worries about monsters attacking his home. However, in contrast to earlier sessions when frightening themes had arisen, Deanna was able to remain regulated, although at times she appeared unsure about how to engage in the play. She was able to stay close to her son, engage with the toys, and respond to questions or suggestions from the clinician in ways that balanced protectiveness with tolerating Brian having control of the play. As her defensive rigidity regarding safety and danger lessened, she found new openness to uncertainty in herself, her children, and the play.

In a session near the end of treatment, Brian had dinosaurs attack the dollhouse while the family slept. Deanna reached for another animal to attack the dinosaurs and keep the family safe, but Brian continued to bring in larger and larger dinosaurs that could mangle any animal Deanna brought to the table. The clinician saw Deanna's frown and furrowed brow and stepped in to offer her support to their joint play, saying "It's scary to see all the big dinosaurs, and we wonder what will happen." With this scaffolding, Deanna was able to tolerate her fears and uncertainty regarding the dangerous play and watched with raised eyebrows while Brian brought the dinosaur smashing down on the playhouse. Aware of the family's impending move, the clinician offered a hopeful narrative for Brian to consider incorporating. The clinician stated, "Even though the big dinosaurs made things so scary, I wonder if the family will keep each other safe?" Brian showed that the family members escaped their collapsing home together. The clinician ended the session by commenting on how very strong and brave the family members were and how very lucky they were to have stayed together even while big things happened around them. Deanna was also able to stay connected with the play; she was a quiet partner but one who was able to take in the same message her son needed to hear; this family could be a source of safety.

The family shared a story at the end of treatment that indicated their developing strengths as parents. The staff at the residence had put a great deal of pressure on Deanna regarding Annie's continued use of a pacifier, insisting it was preventing her language development and needed to be taken from her. They expected Deanna to remove all pacifiers from her room so that Annie would not have access to them. Deanna and Charlie discussed the issue and reported that they felt that Annie used the pacifier to soothe when she was upset or nervous. They made the connections with their own needs to have nondestructive tools to manage difficult feelings and decided that Annie's use of the pacifier was not such a terrible thing. Deanna was angry at the staff for their negative focus on the pacifier but proud that she was able to advocate for her daughter.

TREATMENT COMPLETION

Deanna and her children completed their residential stay and moved with Charlie into a subsidized housing program. The clinician was able to make one transitional visit during which she talked with the family about other available treatment options; however, the family declined further treatment. In reflecting on what she had learned from the CPP sessions, Deanna shared thoughts that seemed to capture the progress she had made during treatment. Deanna reflected, "It's been hard to . . . keep my anger under control sometimes, so having [the clinician] be there and give me advice on how to handle it better has helped. Like, I know how to handle the situations without overreacting now." She went on to describe how these changes had affected her relationship with her children by saying, "Now that I don't overreact as much, [the children] feel like . . . if they do upset me, that it's all right now . . . like instead of having to be perfect."

There were, of course, many unanswered questions as this family terminated treatment. The treatment course had been relatively short given the rapid rate of the children's development and the family's complex history. There were issues left unexplored and unresolved, and the chronic nature of addiction created considerable risk of relapse for one or both parents. As treatment terminated, the clinician and family explored the many ways that the family's narrative might unfold in the future, each path marked by the progress made in treatment, the family's strengths as well as vulnerabilities, and the challenges ahead.

COMMENTARY

The challenges inherent in blending the diverse "cultures" of infant mental health intervention and substance abuse treatment are acknowledged by the authors of this chapter and by others (Bromberg, Backman, Krow, & Fankel,

2010). This case illustrates some of the challenges of delivering CPP in a residential milieu that is focused on helping parents succeed in early recovery from addiction.

When CPP clinicians work within a residential treatment program, they will necessarily interact with treatment milieu staff. This ability to collaborate with other treatment providers is a core competency required of CPP clinicians; however, this task becomes more difficult in a residential setting in which staff need to maintain careful control over the milieu environment and will have ideas and recommendations about who should be included in the treatment. Clinicians must be aware of this difficulty and work particularly hard to ensure that the family's needs and wishes are understood. Supervision is often a useful vehicle for these considerations. In the treatment described here, the clinician states that she "thought carefully with the staff about whom to include in the treatment," and she included the children's father from the outset. Thus it appears that significant weight was given to the wishes of the milieu staff. Giving decision-making authority to the staff is not, however, consistent with CPP. Rather, as the clinician discussed in deciding whether to include the younger daughter in sessions, the CPP clinician generally thinks collaboratively with the caregiver to determine who should be included in treatment. Should the other parent be included? Other children? These questions are discussed with the caregiver during assessment, taking into account issues of safety and the clinical needs of the child and caregiver.

Furthermore, the decision to include the children's father in the treatment had other consequences that affected assessment and intervention. During the assessment, each parent reported having witnessed intimate partner violence throughout their childhoods, placing them at increased risk for violence in their adult relationships. The clinician followed protocol by meeting individually with each parent to privately discuss their own histories. However, the clinician did not note whether she asked the parents about violence within their relationship. It was also not noted if either parent reported being the victim or perpetrator of domestic violence.

Having both caregivers participate in CPP provided opportunities for the children to repair relationships and experience their parents in a state in which they were able to provide adequate care. However, working with two parents also added to the case's complexity. It is possible that, with both parents present during most of the assessment period, they may not have felt comfortable revealing information about sensitive topics such as domestic violence. This may have left the clinician without crucial knowledge about challenges to safety in the parents' relationship and about a traumatic stressor to which the children may have been exposed.

The clinician's reflections on the critically important fact that "emotionally difficult material that will necessarily be raised during child–parent work could become a trigger for relapse" may have led to her apparent decision not to include 4-year-old Brian's traumatic experiences with his parents as part of the narrative developed in the treatment. The need to work actively to avoid relapse is one of the major challenges in adapting CPP for use with families with addictions. In this case, the clinician notes that both parents described their separation from their children and the children's placement in foster care as among their most devastating experiences. We wonder whether the clinician's laudable wish to help the parents avoid relapse may have been behind her focus on themes of loss and separation in Brian's play as well as her statement that she understood Brian as "making sense of parents who, now sober, probably seemed quite different from the parents [he] had come to know, *however briefly*, in their earlier time together" (emphasis added). In fact, Brian was in foster care for about 6 months. He lived for the first 3 years of his life with parents who described themselves as difficult to rouse, sometimes unconscious, ill when they were not high, and coming and going, in the father's case, from episodes in rehabilitation centers or in jail. CPP, as it was conceived, developed, and tested, would have helped Brian and his parents create a joint narrative to communicate and make meaning of Brian's long experience of living with parents who were unresponsive to him and may, on occasion, have appeared to be dead. It seems likely that the clinician's realistic concerns about the possibility of relapse may have led her to focus instead on the experience of loss surrounding Brian's time in foster care, because that experience resonated with the parents' senses of what had been devastating in their own lives.

In spite of these challenges to fidelity during the treatment process, much about the intervention described in this chapter is classic CPP, beautifully delivered. The careful assessment, the focus on understanding the parents' trauma histories as well as their memories of angels in their nurseries, the explicit and patient work to help the parents more effectively observe and understand their children, the holding of the mother's emotional response to her children's play, and the use of play to help the parent and the clinician build a joint understanding of the child's internal world are all hallmarks of CPP. The clinician was extremely sensitive in reflecting on the discrepancies between what Brian was ready to express and what his parents were ready to understand in timing her interventions. This balance of the parents' and the child's needs embodies the CPP value of holding both the parent and child in mind when intervening. Indeed, given the vulnerability of parents in early stages of recovery from addiction, this empathic holding of the parent's experience is essential to work with this population.

The fact that so much changed for this family, and in such positive ways, is testimony to CPP's efficacy, or at least this clinician's efficacy, in their lives. It seems clear that it is possible to successfully use CPP interventions in a residential substance abuse treatment program by helping parents and children understand and reflect on themselves and on one another. This chapter confirms our clinical experience that, despite the struggles associated with changing deep–seated patterns of addiction, there is nothing about early recovery per se that prevents parents from dividing their attention and making space to understand their children's internal worlds and meet their children's needs.

This case study demonstrates that (1) CPP clinicians are at risk for elevating the demands of a treatment milieu over CPP's demands that clinical decisions be made in collaboration with the caregiver and (2) clinical concerns that negative affects arising in a CPP session will become relapse triggers may compel a clinician, either unconsciously or after due deliberation, to avoid a full exploration of the child's traumatic experiences. Fortunately, this case also demonstrates that even should clinicians trip, unwittingly or purposefully, into pitfalls to CPP fidelity, the intervention can bring great benefits to both recovering parents and their children.

ACKNOWLEDGMENTS

The treatment described in this chapter was provided as part of Project BRIGHT, a Substance Abuse and Mental Health Service–funded intervention (No. 1U79SM059460-01) provided by a partnership between the Institute for Health and Recovery and Jewish Family and Children's Service, in Massachusetts. We would like to thank Norma Finkelstein, PhD, the other clinicians and project staff, the project evaluation team at Boston University, led by Ruth Paris, PhD, and the families from whom we learned so much. In particular, we are grateful to Deanna and her family for sharing the work described here.

REFERENCES

Borelli, J. L., West, J. L., DeCoste, C., & Suchman, N. E. (2012). Emotionally avoidant language in the parenting interviews of substance-dependent mothers: Associations with reflective functioning, recent substance use, and parenting behavior. *Infant Mental Health Journal, 33*(5), 506–519.

Bromberg, S. R., Backman, T. L., Krow, J., & Frankel, K. A. (2010). The Haven Mother's House Modified Therapeutic Community: Mending the gap in infant mental health services for pregnant and parenting mothers with drug addiction. *Infant Mental Health Journal, 31,* 255–276.

Fivaz-Depeursinge, E., Corboz-Warnery, A., & Keren, M. (2004). The primary triangle: Treating infants in their families. In A.J. Sameroff, S.C. McDonough, & K.L Rosenblum (Eds.), *Treating parent–infant relationship problems. Strategies for intervention.* New York: Guilford Press.

Fraiberg, S., Adelson, E., & Shapiro, V. (1975). Ghosts in the nursery: A psychoanalytic approach to the problems of impaired infant–mother relationships. *Journal of the American Academy of Child Psychiatry, 14*(3), 387–421.

Lieberman, A. F., Padrón, E., Van Horn, P., & Harris, W. W. (2005). Angels in the nursery: The intergenerational transmission of benevolent parental influences. *Infant Mental Health Journal, 26*(6), 504–520.

Lieberman, A. F., & Van Horn, P. (2005). *Don't hit my mommy!: A manual for child–parent psychotherapy with young witnesses of family violence.* Washington, DC: Zero to Three.

Lieberman, A. F., & Van Horn, P. (2008). *Psychotherapy with infants and young children: Repairing the effects of stress and trauma on early attachment.* New York: Guilford Press.

Pajulo, M., Suchman, N., Kalland, M., & Mayes, L. (2006). Enhancing the effectiveness of residential treatment for substance abusing pregnant and parenting women: Focus on maternal reflective functioning and mother–child relationship. *Infant Mental Health Journal, 27*(5), 448–465.

Suchman, N. E., DeCoste, C., Leigh, D., & Borelli, J. (2010). Reflective functioning in mothers with drug use disorders: Implications for dyadic interactions with infants and toddlers. *Attachment and Human Development, 12*(6), 567–585.

PART IV

PARENT–CHILD INTERACTION THERAPY (PCIT)

9

Parent–Child Interaction Therapy

An Overview

Joaquin Borrego, Jr., Chelsea Klinkebiel,
and Alexandra Gibson

Parent–child interaction therapy (PCIT) is an evidence-based behavioral parent training intervention that was originally developed by Sheila Eyberg for families with young children displaying socially disruptive behavior problems, such as physical aggression and noncompliance (McNeil & Hembree-Kigin, 2010). Most of the empirical work on PCIT has focused on young children with externalizing behavior problems between the ages of 2 and 7 (Bell & Eyberg, 2002); however, PCIT has been increasingly applied with different treatment and demographic populations. For instance, the past 10 to 15 years have seen increased attention given to the applicability of PCIT in changing the parenting styles and techniques of physically abusive caregivers and improving the parent–child relationships in these cases.

THEORETICAL RATIONALE

Parenting research shows that an authoritative parenting style provides the greatest potential for optimal child outcomes (Baumrind, 1967). Parents who can sustain a balance of providing warmth and support for their child while maintaining a high standard of expected behavior typically have more functional relationships than those caregivers with maladaptive parent–child relationships and poor behavior management skills (Kaufmann et al., 2000).

Behavioral parenting therapies, such as PCIT, can be utilized to improve a parent's behavior management skills as well as enhance the relationship between the parent and the child.

The concept of successfully creating a secure, positive parent–child relationship while simultaneously providing appropriate limits is based on attachment theory, which postulates that a stable parent–child relationship wherein the child can depend on the caretaker to attend to his or her needs is necessary for positive growth. A maladaptive attachment often leads to decreased social competence and higher levels of problem behaviors, such as aggression (Luycks et al., 2011). Maladaptive attachment is also linked to greater parental stress and child maltreatment (Brinkmeyer & Eyberg, 2003) as well as higher levels of externalizing (e.g., overactivity, impulsivity, aggression) and internalizing behaviors (e.g., depression, social withdrawal) in later childhood (O'Connor, Collins, & Supplee, 2012).

Another theoretical perspective that is important to PCIT is social learning theory, which postulates that children learn within their own social context through processes such as modeling and observation. More specifically, there are environmental contingencies that help shape functional and dysfunctional behavior (Bell & Eyberg, 2002). Patterson's (1982) coercive cycle of dysfunctional parent–child interactions, in which the parent–child relationship is influenced by escalating aversive behaviors as the parent and child both attempt to gain control of the situation, is useful in helping explain the development and maintenance of maladaptive child and parent behaviors. Patterson's coercive model can be understood from a social learning perspective (Brinkmeyer & Eyberg, 2003). A parent positively reinforces a child's attention-seeking behavior (e.g., whining) with attention (e.g., yelling); however, the parent providing attention to the child is negatively reinforced by the child ceasing the aversive behavior. Thus the whining behavior of the child and the yelling behavior of the adult are both reinforced, increasing the likelihood that both will occur again. PCIT can be used to reset this maladaptive reinforcement cycle by teaching parents effective behavior management skills, such as ignoring attention-seeking or disruptive behaviors and praising appropriate behaviors.

TREATMENT THEMES

Emphasis on the Parent–Child Relationship

The general goal of PCIT is to improve the parent–child relationship and dyadic interactions, and this is accomplished through coaching the parent on how to respond to the child during play activities. Related to this goal, the therapist also works on decreasing parent and child problematic behaviors and increasing parent and child positive behaviors. The therapist teaches new, noncoercive skills and/or further refines skills that parents already have in their repertoire. The skills taught are generally focused on increasing the parent's ability to attend to the child in a positive manner and improving the parent's ability to effectively manage the child's problematic behaviors.

Live Coaching of the Parent

PCIT is an intensive intervention in that the PCIT therapist works with both the parent and child, observing the dyad interacting with each other and providing direct instruction and feedback to the parent in real time. Although it is live coaching, most of the PCIT therapist's coaching is conducted behind a one-way mirror while the parent wears a "bug-in-the-ear" hearing device and interacts with the child in a separate room. This aspect of PCIT is unique, as most interventions focus on either the parent or the child in individual therapy or work with the parent in the context of group-based parenting classes. In PCIT, parents get to practice these skills with their children, and the therapist is able to provide immediate feedback and reinforcement.

PROGRAM COMPONENTS AND CHARACTERISTICS

A Two-Stage Model

PCIT is based on the two-stage model developed by Hanf (1969). The two phases of PCIT are the *child-directed interaction* (CDI) stage and the *parent-directed interaction* (PDI) stage. During CDI, parents are first taught to use play skills as a mechanism for change. CDI resembles what some might consider traditional play therapy. Specifically, parents are instructed to allow the child to guide the play and to refrain from providing commands, questions, or criticisms. The goal is to increase the behavior-specific positive praise that the parent provides the child, while simultaneously decreasing attention to negative or disruptive behaviors, such as aggression or whining.

During PDI, parents learn how to employ child behavior management skills to better regulate the child's behaviors. Specific skills include how to appropriately set limits and to provide consistent discipline (Bell & Eyberg, 2002). Progression through and successful completion of PCIT is based on the parent demonstrating mastery of certain parenting skills (this is discussed in more detail later in the chapter). For successful completion, the parent must reach mastery criteria in each of the two treatment phases. PCIT is considered a short-term intervention, and the average length of treatment required to successfully complete both phases is between 11 and 16 sessions (McNeil & Hembree-Kigin, 2010).

CDI Skills

During the first phase of treatment, CDI, parents learn play therapy skills that help them improve the quality of the parent–child relationship. During the first CDI session (CDI didactic), PCIT therapists model attending and reinforcement skills for parents and then ensure the parents understand the concepts by having them demonstrate the skills during role plays. These skills are known as the *PRIDE* skills: Praise, Reflection, Imitation, Description, and Enjoyment.

When teaching *praise*, clinicians encourage parents to attach a label to the praise that describes the specific positive behavior of the child (e.g., "Thank you for sharing the doll" vs. "Thank you"). Praise provides positive reinforcement to the child, and labeled praise allows the child to know the specific behavior that warranted the positive attention. *Reflection* involves repeating or paraphrasing a child's verbalization. This skill is used in order to let the child lead the conversation, to model speech and listening skills, and to increase verbal communication (Eyberg & Funderburk, 2011). Parents are also encouraged to let their child lead the play and show their approval by *imitating* his or her play. By providing a *description* of the child's behavior, parents demonstrate that they are following the child's lead. This skill also helps parents to model good speech and to focus a child's attention on a task (Eyberg & Funderburk, 2011). Finally, parents are encouraged to display their *enjoyment* while playing with a child (e.g., smiling or hugging) to increase the warmth of the interaction. Learning the PRIDE skills not only improves the quality of the parent–child relationship but also increases the amount of social reinforcement parents give to children for positive behaviors. In addition, during the CDI portion of treatment, parents learn to ignore disruptive and negative attention-seeking behaviors (e.g., whining, yelling, and tantrums) in order to stop the cycle of reinforcement for these behaviors and reduce their frequency, a technique often referred to as active ignoring or selective attention.

PDI Skills

After parents have mastered the skills presented in CDI, they move to the second phase of treatment, PDI. In this phase, parents learn how to increase child compliance by using effective commands (e.g., making commands direct, simple, and understandable). In addition, parents learn to use consistent guidelines for determining when a child is compliant or non-compliant. For example, parents learn to give children 5 seconds to comply (or begin to comply) with a command. Parents also learn to use a consistent time-out procedure utilizing a time-out chair and a backup time-out space for cases when a child does not stay in the time-out chair. Parents continue to socially reinforce prosocial behaviors, but now use a defined time-out procedure for negative behaviors (e.g., defiance, noncompliance, physical aggression).

In PCIT, time-out is performed by having a child sit in a time-out chair in the corner of the room for 3 minutes plus 5 seconds of quiet (Eyberg & Funderburk, 2011). Parents use active ignoring while the child sits in the time-out chair, and the child gets to rejoin the play once he or she completes the allotted time and complies with the original command. When children leave the chair before the 3 minutes is up or engage in unsafe behaviors in the chair (e.g., standing on or rocking the chair), they go to time-out in a backup area that serves to keep the child safe, but remove any potential reinforcement (e.g., a small room or cubicle that is free of objects). Children stay in the backup area for 1 minute (plus 5 seconds of quiet), and then return to the time-out chair for 3 minutes plus 5 seconds of quiet, getting out of the time-out chair once they comply with the original command. When a time-out chair or backup area is not feasible at home, parents may be coached in the use of a *swoop and go* technique in which toys are cleaned up quickly and the child is left alone in the empty room for the allotted time (McNeil & Hembree-Kigin, 2010).

As with CDI, when parents begin PDI, they first attend a session without the child. In the session the therapist models the new skills and role-plays with parents to ensure their understanding (PDI didactic). During the first PDI session with the child present, the new procedure is explained to him or her before it is implemented. A common procedure in many agencies is to use a stuffed bear to model the time-out procedure for children in an unintimidating way. In this procedure, the therapist plays with "Mr. Bear," giving him commands as they play. When Mr. Bear is noncompliant, he sits in the time-out chair, and when he is compliant, he receives labeled praises. The complete time-out procedure, including the time-out room, is demonstrated for children with Mr. Bear before parents implement it with their children.

Assessment in PCIT

Assessment is an integral part of PCIT, and multiple modes of assessment are used to guide treatment. All parents complete a pretreatment assessment session consisting of various self-report measures and a behavioral observation. In addition to a clinical interview, parents complete a measure of child externalizing behavior, the Eyberg Child Behavior Inventory (ECBI; Eyberg & Pincus, 1999). If a child is attending preschool or school, the child's primary teacher also completes the Sutter–Eyberg Student Behavior Inventory—Revised (SESBI-R; Eyberg & Pincus, 1999), a measure of child externalizing behavior similar to the ECBI. Parents may also complete a broadband scale of child psychopathology such as the Child Behavior Checklist (CBCL; Achenbach & Rescorla, 2001) or the Behavior Assessment Scale for Children (BASC; Reynolds & Kamphaus, 2004), especially if there are concerns about other problems such as internalizing symptoms (McNeil & Hembree-Kigin, 2010).

In addition to child functioning, pretreatment assessment may include measures of parental functioning with regard to stress and psychological symptoms. Common measures include the Parenting Stress Index (PSI; Abidin, 1990) and measures of parental depression, such as the Beck Depression Inventory (BDI; Beck, Ward, Mendelson, Mock, & Erbaugh, 1961; Beck, Steer, & Brown, 1996) and the Center for Epidemiologic Studies Depression Scale (CES-D; Radloff, 1977). Other common self-report measures completed by parents at pretreatment include the Child Abuse Potential Inventory (CAPI; Milner, 1994; Ondersma, Chaffin, Mullins, & LeBreton, 2005) and the Child Rearing Inventory (CRI; Brestan, Eyberg, Algina, Johnson, & Boggs, 2003). The battery of self-report assessments in PCIT is considered flexible to allow for individualized assessment for each family (McNeil & Hembree-Kigin, 2010).

Along with these self-report measures, each parent–child dyad completes a behavioral observation. This observation is divided into three separate, 5-minute coding situations: Child-Led Play, Parent-Led Play, and Cleanup. During Child-Led Play, parents are instructed to let the child play with whatever toys he or she wishes and to follow the child's lead, while in Parent-Led Play, parents are instructed to choose the activity and get the child to follow their lead and rules (Eyberg & Funderburk, 2011). Finally, in Cleanup, parents are instructed to have the child clean up all of the toys in the room by him- or herself. During the three situations, behaviors of parents and children are coded by the clinician using the Dyadic Parent–Child Interaction Coding System—Fourth Edition (DPICS), a coding system that includes codes for parent and child verbalizations, vocalizations, and physical behaviors (Eyberg, Nelson, Ginn, Bhuiyan, & Boggs, 2013).

The assessment battery completed at pretreatment is repeated after completion of the PDI phase (posttreatment). A key component of PCIT, however, is ongoing assessment throughout treatment. Parents continue to complete the ECBI at the beginning of each treatment session in order to monitor the frequency of child externalizing behavior problems. Also at the beginning of each treatment session parents are coded using the DPICS to ascertain their use of PCIT skills while playing with the child during a 5-minute observation period. This short behavioral observation allows therapists to determine how well parents are learning and increasing their use of skills as well as areas for improvement.

Format of Treatment Sessions

Once the pretreatment assessment session is completed, therapists conduct the CDI didactic, meeting with parents alone in order to orient them to PCIT and to teach them the skills utilized in CDI. Meeting without the child present allows therapists to discuss the skills with parents, answer questions, and help parents to problem-solve how the skills can be used with their children. During this didactic session, therapists present the skills to parents; however, parents also actively practice using the skills with the therapist before implementing them with the referred child.

After the CDI didactic session, parents complete CDI skills coaching sessions. As described earlier, each coaching session begins with a 5-minute coding period in which each parent is observed interacting with the child. However, most of the treatment session is devoted to therapists live coaching the parents. During coaching, therapists encourage the use of PRIDE skills by having parents repeat their verbal prompts and praising parents' use of the skills. In order to achieve mastery in CDI, parents must give 10 labeled praises, 10 reflections, and 10 behavior descriptions during the 5-minute coding period that begins each session.

The next phase of treatment begins with another didactic session (PDI didactic) in which parents learn about and practice using effective commands. They also practice the time-out procedure by walking through each step with therapists. During PDI coaching sessions, parents are again coded at the beginning of the session in their skill usage, with most of the treatment session devoted to coaching. Mastery of PDI skills is reached when 75% of the commands parents give to children are direct commands, and parents respond correctly to child behavior (e.g., labeled praise for compliance or time-out for noncompliance) 75% of the time during coding.

Resources and Equipment

Treatment with PCIT involves several standard spaces and types of equipment. Coaching is provided from behind a one-way mirror, with the parent and child in the playroom and the therapist(s) in an observation room. The parent wears a "bug-in-the-ear" speaker device so that therapists can speak directly to them. Commonly used devices include Bluetooth headsets, but may include less expensive two-way radios with earpieces. In agencies where out-of-room coaching is not possible owing to the lack of an observation room, in-room coaching may be utilized, in which therapists stand behind parents or sit unobtrusively in the room to provide feedback. Although this can make coaching more feasible for some organizations, it can present challenges, such as confusing the child about whom they should interact with as well as undermining parental authority (McNeil & Hembree-Kigin, 2010). In addition to the playroom and observation room, a backup time-out area is used. This time-out area can be a separate room or an enclosed area of the playroom and should not contain any furniture or other items.

Given that PCIT is centered on play between a child and parent, preferred toys are used to encourage interaction by the dyad. Toys that promote creative and constructive play are recommended (e.g., blocks, play food, dollhouses, crayons and paper), while toys that encourage aggressive play are discouraged (e.g., balls, toy guns, action figures; Eyberg & Funderburk, 2011). Toys that may require parents to set limits or take over the play (e.g., painting, games with rules) and toys that do not encourage verbal interaction (e.g., books and video games) are also discouraged.

RESEARCH EVIDENCE FOR PCIT

Overview

As noted above, PCIT is an evidence-based treatment that accompanies a variety of treatment populations and has accumulated a substantial body of empirical support. Not only are reductions in socially disruptive behaviors observed at home and in clinical settings, but treatment gains from PCIT generalized to school settings are demonstrated (Funderburk et al., 1998; McNeil, Eyberg, Hembree-Eisenstadt, Newcomb, & Funderburk, 1991; Schuhmann, Foote, Eyberg, Boggs, & Algina, 1998). In addition, studies suggest that treatment gains are maintained over a significant period of time, ranging from 1 year (Eyberg et al., 2001) to 6 years posttreatment (Hood & Eyberg, 2003).

Successful application of PCIT has occurred with a variety of different populations, including ethnic minorities (e.g., Borrego, Anhalt, Terao, Vargas, & Urquiza, 2006; Capage, Bennett, & McNeil, 2001; McCabe & Yeh, 2009), international families (e.g., Leung, Tsang, Heung, & Yiu, 2009; Matos, Torres, Santiago, Jurado, & Rodríguez, 2006), and children with developmental disabilities (Bagner & Eyberg, 2007). Adaptations of PCIT have been developed for use in a group format (Niec, Hemme, Yopp, & Brestan, 2005), as well as for behavior problems associated with a variety of other phenomena, including chronic illness (Bagner, Fernandez, & Eyberg, 2004), separation anxiety (Choate, Pincus, Eyberg, & Barlow, 2005; Pincus, Santucci, Ehrenreich, & Eyberg, 2008), and attention-deficit/hyperactivity disorder (Nixon, 2001). Studies of PCIT suggest high caregiver satisfaction with the treatment (Brestan, Jacobs, Rayfield, & Eyberg, 1999) and the generalization of techniques to other children (e.g., untreated siblings; Brestan, Eyberg, Boggs, & Algina, 1997).

PCIT is shown to have a positive impact on the caregivers' functioning and their behaviors exhibited in session. For instance, PCIT was found to reduce parents' depressive symptoms (e.g., Timmer et al., 2011) and increase their locus of control (Hood & Eyberg, 2003). Importantly, parents participating in PCIT report lower abuse potential at the conclusion of therapy (e.g., Borrego, Urquiza, Rasmussen, & Zebell, 1999) along with a decrease in distress (e.g., Timmer, Urquiza, Zebell, & McGrath, 2005). Related to specific parental behaviors, PCIT is shown to increase prosocial behaviors (e.g., verbal praises; Thomas & Zimmer-Gembeck, 2012) and to decrease negative behaviors (e.g., questions and criticisms; Eisenstadt, Eyberg, McNeil, Newcomb, & Funderburk, 1993).

When examining treatment outcomes, it is important to consider factors that may lead families to not experience the full benefit of interventions or to drop out of treatment. Recent research has identified some factors that may put families at risk for attrition. These include young maternal age (Werba, Eyberg, Boggs, & Algina, 2006), low family income (Lanier et al., 2011), and ethnic minority status (Bagner & Graziano, 2013). Less successful treatment outcomes for families who complete PCIT are shown to be related to higher levels of parenting stress and lower parental education (Bagner & Graziano, 2013; Werba et al., 2006), as well as child characteristics such as callous–unemotional traits (Kimonis, Bagner, Linares, Blake, & Rodriguez, 2013). Therefore, clinicians should assess for various risk factors within families that may lead to attrition, lower attendance, less adherence, and lower acceptability of treatment. When these risk factors are identified, steps should be taken to reduce their impact.

PCIT and Family Violence

Although there are substantial data to support the efficacy of PCIT with different populations, there was previously an absence in the literature regarding the applicability of PCIT with abusive families. Urquiza and McNeil's (1996) proposal that PCIT could be used with physically abusive families is based on the premise that a social learning perspective could help account for the development and maintenance of physically abusive parent–child relationships. In their conceptual article, the authors highlighted Gerald Patterson's (1982) social learning framework to help explain physically abusive parent–child relationships. The authors argued that Patterson's description of the coercive cycle in explaining the development and maintenance of child behavior problems, in general, can be applied in the context of examining physically abusive parent–child relationships. More specifically, Urquiza and McNeil proposed that physically abusive parents use violence (e.g., hitting) to get the child to stop engaging in aversive behaviors (e.g., whining, crying) or to get them to comply with a command. Observational data of physically abusive parent–child dyads provide support for targeting specific parenting behaviors in PCIT (Borrego, Timmer, Urquiza, & Follette, 2004; Hakman, Chaffin, Funderburk, & Silovsky, 2009; Timmer, Borrego, & Urquiza, 2002).

One of the first published studies with this population was a single-case design examining PCIT with a mother considered to be at risk for child physical abuse (Borrego et al., 1999). The mother was considered at risk because she called in crisis, had a previous history of CPS involvement, had a child with an intellectual disability and fetal alcohol syndrome, and reported that the child had behavior problems. Data from standardized measures the mother completed suggested that PCIT was effective in reducing her child abuse potential and stress related to parenting, as well as the number and intensity of the child's behavior problems. Observations of the mother–child dyad through treatment showed that the mother increased the frequency with which she used verbal praise and descriptions (thus positively attending to the child more) and decreased her use of asking the child questions.

In a similar study, Timmer and colleagues (Timmer, Urquiza, Herschell, et al., 2006) used a single-case design to examine the effectiveness of PCIT with a foster-adoptive parent caring for a child with a history of maltreatment and displaying physical aggression. Like the Borrego et al. (1999) study, there was a decrease in child behavior problems and parenting stress and an increase of parent verbal praise after completing PCIT.

Larger studies have focused on the usefulness of PCIT with families involved in the child welfare system. In a randomized trial involving 110 physically abusive parents, Chaffin and colleagues (Chaffin et al., 2004) compared PCIT to a standard community-based parenting program (i.e., parenting classes). The data from this randomized trial suggested that standard PCIT was effective in reducing negative parent behaviors. In addition to this outcome, at a median follow-up of 850 days (2+ years), only 19% of parents who participated in PCIT were reinvestigated for child physical abuse, compared to 49% of parents who participated in the community-based group program. These findings are significant as they highlight that PCIT is effective with families involved in the child welfare system for child physical abuse. In a similar study with 192 parents referred by the child welfare system, Chaffin and colleagues (Chaffin, Funderburk, Bard, Valle, & Gurwich, 2011) found that a combined motivational enhancement plus PCIT package reduced child welfare recidivism when compared to services as usual. This study replicated previous laboratory results (Chaffin et al., 2004) in a field implementation trial.

Timmer and colleagues (Timmer et al., 2005; Timmer, Urquiza, & Zebell, 2006) examined the effectiveness of PCIT with families participating in the child welfare system. In one study, the authors examined the effectiveness of PCIT with 136 biological parent–child dyads with 91 of these children having a history of child maltreatment (Timmer et al., 2005). Of the 91 children with a history of maltreatment, 59 of the parents were the maltreating parent. Outcomes of this study showed that PCIT was effective in reducing child behavior problems, parent distress, and risk for abuse. In a similar outcome study, Timmer, Urquiza, and Zebell (2006) examined the effectiveness of PCIT with children in foster care. In this study, 75 nonabusive, foster parent–child dyads were compared to 98 nonabusive biological parent–child dyads. Both groups showed an improvement in child behavior problems and caregiver distress with no differences in treatment outcome between the two groups. Studies similar to the ones by Chaffin and colleagues and Timmer and colleagues were conducted in Australia with similar results (Thomas & Zimmer-Gembeck, 2011, 2012).

More recent attention has focused on other forms of interpersonal family violence, such as domestic violence. Borrego, Gutow, Reicher, and Barker (2008) proposed that PCIT also can be applied with families that have experienced domestic violence. The authors highlight the effects that domestic violence can have on the family, the children, and the parent–child relationship. A study by Timmer, Ware, Urquiza, and Zebell (2010) compared children who were maltreated and exposed to interpersonal violence (IPV) to children who were clinic-referred for maltreatment, but not exposed to IPV. The results of the study suggested that PCIT can be effective in reducing child behavior problems and caregivers' level of psychological distress in cases of child maltreatment and/or IPV.

In summary, the available data for the effectiveness of PCIT with families who have experienced family violence (i.e., child physical abuse, domestic violence) suggest that PCIT can be effective in reducing child behavior problems, child abuse potential, and caregivers' psychological distress. The data also suggest that PCIT can be effective in reducing negative parenting behaviors and increasing prosocial parent behaviors (e.g., verbal praises). Although no published studies have documented the effectiveness of PCIT with other forms of child abuse (e.g., child sexual abuse), recent conceptual writings have focused on the potential applicability of PCIT in cases in which sexual abuse has occurred (Urquiza & Blacker, 2012).

CULTURAL CONSIDERATIONS

As with other types of psychosocial interventions (Zayas, Borrego, & Domenech-Rodriquez, 2009), criticism that cultural factors are often overlooked in treatment delivery has resulted in increased attention to cultural variables in PCIT (Anhalt & Borrego, 2010; Butler & Eyberg, 2006).

PCIT researchers have attempted to address this concern in the context of services. This ranges from recommendations on how to address cultural factors in PCIT to cultural adaptations of PCIT for specific groups (Barker, Cook, & Borrego, 2010). Some researchers have directly examined the effectiveness of standard PCIT with different ethnic/racial minority groups. For instance, PCIT was examined with African American families in a series of studies, and favorable outcomes were observed (Capage et al., 2001; Fernandez, Butler, & Eyberg, 2011).

One noteworthy cultural adaptation is Bigfoot and Funderburk's (2011) adapted PCIT for use with American Indian and Native American families. The model, Honoring Children, Making Relatives, embeds the basic tenets and treatment components of PCIT within a framework that focuses on traditional American Indian and Alaskan Native beliefs and parenting practices. Although guidelines are provided, treatment outcome data are not available regarding the cultural adaptation of PCIT for this target population.

Some PCIT treatment outcome data for families of Latino origin is available. The first published outcome study of PCIT in Spanish was conducted by Borrego and colleagues (2006). This study showed that a basic translation of PCIT in Spanish was effective in bringing about change in a parent–child dyad. Since that publication, other treatment researchers have spent considerable time making thoughtful adaptations for other Latino-origin groups. Treatment adaptations by Maribel Matos for families living in Puerto Rico (Matos, Bauermeister, & Bernal, 2009; Matos et al., 2006) and Kristen McCabe for Mexican American families living in southern California (McCabe & Yeh, 2009; McCabe, Yeh, Garland, Lau, & Chavez, 2005; McCabe, Yeh, Lau, & Argote, 2012) have produced favorable treatment outcomes. Kristen McCabe's research includes one of the few treatment outcome studies that has directly compared a standard intervention, in this case PCIT, to a culturally adapted version (i.e., PCIT for Mexican Americans, *Guiando a Niños Activos,* or Guiding Active Children; McCabe & Yeh, 2009). Results suggested that culturally adapted PCIT can be as effective as standard PCIT in reducing child behavior problems. In summary, promising data suggest that both standard PCIT and culturally adapted PCIT can be effective with ethnic and racial minority groups.

TRAINING PROGRAMS AND RESOURCES

The standards for PCIT therapist qualifications were recently updated and published by PCIT International. A comprehensive list of PCIT International training guidelines can be found at *www.pcit.org/training-guidelines.* In addition, for a full list of PCIT master trainers and contact information for training sites, see the PCIT International website at *www.pcit.org.*

To become a certified PCIT therapist, clinicians are required to hold at least a master's degree in a mental health-related field and be independently licensed or working under the license of another mental health provider. PCIT-specific training requirements include 40 hours of face-to-face training with an approved PCIT trainer (10 hours of this training may occur through online education), a minimum of twice-monthly supervision and consultation with the trainer, and having treatment sessions reviewed by the trainer. Therapist acquisition of the PCIT skills will be assessed by the trainer, and therapists must complete at least two full PCIT protocols/cases prior to certification.

CONCLUSIONS

PCIT is an effective parent training intervention for families of young children with significant behavior problems. A wealth of literature supports its efficacy in reducing disruptive child behavior problems, parenting distress, and risk for abuse, as well as improving the quality of parent–child relationships. Although PCIT is a standardized parent training intervention, it has been adapted in many ways to provide treatment that is culturally appropriate and acceptable. Mental health practitioners and mental health service administrators should be encouraged by findings that PCIT is an evidence-based treatment that can be useful in working with families with a history of interpersonal family violence, including physical abuse and domestic violence.

SUGGESTED RESOURCES

Books

- McNeil, C. B., & Hembree-Kigin, T. L. (2010). *Parent–child interaction therapy* (2nd ed.). New York: Springer.

Websites

- PCIT International
  www.pcit.org

- UC Davis PCIT Training Center
  http://pcit.ucdavis.edu

- UC Davis PCIT for Traumatized Children
  http://pcit.ucdavis.edu/pcit-web-course

  This Web-based training course describes an adaptation of PCIT that was developed specifically for clinicians who are interested in delivering PCIT to maltreated children, traumatized children, and clinicians/families involved in the child welfare system.

Other Resources

- Eyberg, S. M., & Funderburk, B. (2011). *Parent–child interaction therapy protocol*
  www.pcit.org/web-store

- PCIT Listserv
  http://pcit.ucdavis.edu/resources/join-listserv

REFERENCES

Abidin, R. R. (1990). *Parenting Stress Index/Short Form*. Lutz, FL: Psychological Assessment Resources.

Achenbach, T. M., & Rescorla, L. (2000). *Manual for the ASEBA preschool forms and profiles*. Burlington: University of Vermont Department of Psychiatry, Research Center for Children, Youth, and Families.

Anhalt, K. & Borrego, Jr., J. (2010). Cultural issues in PCIT. In C. B. McNeil & T. Hembree-Kigin (Eds.), *Parent–child interaction therapy* (2nd ed.). New York: Springer.

Bagner, D. M., & Eyberg, S. M. (2007). Parent–child interaction therapy for disruptive behavior in children with mental retardation: A randomized controlled trial. *Journal of Clinical Child and Adolescent Psychology, 36*, 418–429.

Bagner, D. M., Fernandez, M. A., & Eyberg, S. M. (2004). Parent–child interaction therapy and chronic illness: A case study. *Journal of Clinical Psychology in Medical Settings, 11*, 1–6.

Bagner, D. M., & Graziano, P. A. (2013). Barriers to success in parent training for young children with developmental delay: The role of cumulative risk. *Behavior Modification, 37*, 356–377.

Barker, C. H., Cook, K., & Borrego, J. Jr. (2010). Addressing cultural variables in parent training programs with Latino families. *Cognitive and Behavioral Practice, 17*, 157–166.

Baumrind, D. (1967). Child care practices anteceding three patterns of preschool behavior. *Genetic Psychology Monographs, 75*, 43–88.

Beck, A. T., Steer, R. A., & Brown, G. K. (1996). *Manual for the Beck Depression Inventory–II*. San Antonio: Psychological Corporation.

Beck, A. T., Ward, C. H., Mendelson, M., Mock, J., & Erbaugh, J. (1961). An inventory for measuring depression. *Archives of General Psychiatry, 4*, 561–571.

Bell, S., & Eyberg, S. M. (2002). Parent–child interaction therapy. In L. VandeCreek, S. Knapp, & T. L. Jackson (Eds.), *Innovations in Clinical Practice: A Source Book* (Vol. 20). Sarasota, FL: Professional Resource Press.

Bigfoot, D. S., & Funderburk, B. W. (2011). Honoring children, making relatives: The cultural translation of parent–child interaction therapy for American Indian and Native Alaskan families. *Journal of Psychoactive Drugs, 43*, 309–318.

Borrego, J., Anhalt, K., Terao, S. Y., Vargas, E. C., & Urquiza, A. J. (2006). Parent–child interaction therapy with a Spanish-speaking family. *Cognitive and Behavioral Practice, 13*(2), 121–133.

Borrego, J., Jr., Gutow, M. R., Reicher, S., & Barker, C. H. (2008). Parent–child interaction therapy with domestic violence populations. *Journal of Family Violence 23*, 495–505.

Borrego, J., Jr., Timmer, S. G., Urquiza, A. J., & Follette, W. C. (2004). Physically abusive mothers' responses following episodes of child noncompliance and compliance. *Journal of Consulting and Clinical Psychology, 72*(5), 897–903.

Borrego, J., Jr., Urquiza, A. J., Rasmussen, R. A., & Zebell, N. (1999). Parent–child interaction therapy with a family at high risk for physical abuse. *Child Maltreatment, 4*(4), 331–342.

Brestan, E. V., Eyberg, S. M., Algina, J., Johnson, S. B., & Boggs, S. R. (2003). How annoying is it?: Defining parental tolerance for child misbehavior. *Child and Family Behavior Therapy, 25*, 1–15.

Brestan, E. V., Eyberg, S. M., Boggs, S. R., & Algina, J. (1997). Parent–child interaction therapy: Parent perceptions of untreated siblings. *Child and Family Behavior Therapy, 19*, 13–28.

Brestan, E. V., Jacobs, J. R., Rayfield, A. D., & Eyberg, S. M. (1999). A consumer satisfaction measure for parent–child treatments and its relations to measures of child behavior change. *Behavior Therapy, 30*, 17–30.

Brinkmeyer, M. Y., & Eyberg, S. M. (2003). Parent–child interaction therapy for oppositional children. In A. E. Kazdin & J. R. Weisz (Eds.), *Evidence-based psychotherapies for children and adolescents*. New York: Guilford Press.

Butler, A. M., & Eyberg, S. M. (2006). Parent–child interaction therapy and ethnic minority children. *Vulnerable Children and Youth Studies, 1*(3), 246–255.

Capage, L. C., Bennett, G. M., & McNeil, C. B. (2001). A comparison between African American and Caucasian children referred from treatment of disruptive behavior disorders. *Child and Family Behavior Therapy, 23*(1), 1–14.

Chaffin, M., Funderburk, B., Bard, D., Valle, L.A., & Gurwich, R. (2011). A combined motivation and parent–child interaction therapy package reduces child welfare recidivism in a randomized dismantling field trial. *Journal of Consulting and Clinical Psychology, 79*(1), 84–95.

Chaffin, M., Silovsky, J. F., Funderburk, B., Valle, L., Brestan, E. V., Balachova, T., et al., (2004). Parent–child interaction therapy with physically abusive parents: Efficacy for reducing future abuse reports. *Journal of Consulting and Clinical Psychology, 72*(3), 500–510.

Choate, M. L., Pincus, D. B., Eyberg, S. M., & Barlow, D. H. (2005). Parent–child interaction therapy for treatment of separation anxiety disorder in young children: A pilot study. *Cognitive and Behavioral Practice, 12*, 126–135.

Eisenstadt, T. H., Eyberg, S., McNeil, C. B., Newcomb, K., & Funderburk, B. (1993). Parent–child interaction therapy with behavior problem children: Relative effectiveness of two stages and overall treatment outcomes. *Journal of Clinical Child Psychology, 22*, 42–51.

Eyberg, S. M., & Funderburk, B. (2011). *Parent–child interaction therapy protocol*. Gainesville, FL: PCIT International.

Eyberg, S. M., Funderburk, B. W., Hembree-Kigin, T. L., McNeil, C. B., Querido, J. G., & Hood, K. (2001). Parent–child interaction therapy with behavior problem children: One and two year maintenance of treatment effects in the family. *Child and Family Behavior Therapy, 23*, 1–20.

Eyberg, S. M., Nelson, M. M., Ginn, N., Bhuiyan, N., & Boggs, S. R. (2013). *Manual for the dyadic parent–child coding system* (4th ed.). Gainesville, FL: PCIT International.

Eyberg, S. M., & Pincus, D. (1999). *Eyberg Child Behavior Inventory and Sutter–Eyberg Student Behavior Inventory: Professional Manual*. Odessa, FL: Psychological Assessment Resources.

Fernandez, M. A, Butler, A. M., & Eyberg, S. M. (2011). Treatment outcome for low socioeconomic status African American families in parent–child interaction therapy: A pilot study. *Child and Family Behavior Therapy, 33*(1), 32–48.

Funderburk, B. W., Eyberg, S. M., Newcomb, K., McNeil, C., Hembree-Kigin, T., & Capage, L. (1998). Parent–child interaction therapy with behavior problem children: Maintenance of treatment effects in the school setting. *Child and Family Behavior Therapy, 20,* 17–38.

Hakman, M., Chaffin, M., Funderburk, B., & Silovsky, J. (2009). Change trajectories for parent–child interaction sequences during parent–child interaction therapy for child physical abuse. *Child Abuse and Neglect, 33,* 461–470.

Hanf, C. A. (1969). *A two-stage program for modifying maternal controlling during mother–child (M-C) interaction.* Paper presented at the meeting of the Western Psychological Association, Vancouver.

Hood, K. K., & Eyberg, S. M. (2003). Outcomes of parent–child interaction therapy: Mothers' reports of maintenance three to six years after treatment. *Journal of Clinical Child and Adolescent Psychology, 32,* 419–429.

Kaufmann, D., Gesten, E., Santa Lucia, R. C., Salcedo, O., Rendina-Gobioff, G., & Gadd, R. (2000). The relationship between parenting style and children's adjustment: The parent's perspective. *Journal of Child and Family Studies, 9*(2), 231–245.

Kimonis, E. R., Bagner, D. M., Linares, D., Blake, C. A., & Rodriguez, G. (2013). Parent training outcomes among young children with callous-unemotional conduct problems with or at risk for developmental delay. *Journal of Child and Family Studies,* 1–12.

Lanier, P., Kohl, P. L., Benz, J., Swinger, D., Moussette, P., & Drake, B. (2011). Parent–child interaction therapy in a community setting: Examining outcomes, attrition, and treatment setting. *Research on Social Work Practice, 21,* 689–698.

Leung, C., Tsang, S., Heung, K., & Yiu, I. (2009). Effectiveness of parent–child interaction therapy among Chinese families. *Research on Social Work Practice, 19*(3), 304–313.

Luyckx, K., Tildesley, E. A., Soenens, B., Andrews, J. A., Hampson, S. E., Peterson, M., et al. (2011). Parenting and trajectories of children's maladaptive behaviors: A 12-year prospective community study. *Journal of Clinical Child and Adolescent Psychology, 40*(3), 468–478.

Matos, M., Bauermeister, J. J., & Bernal, G. (2009). Parent–child interaction therapy for Puerto Rican preschool children with ADHD and behavior problems: A pilot efficacy study. *Family Process, 48,* 232–252.

Matos, M., Torres, R., Santiago, R., Jurado, M., & Rodríguez, I. (2006). Adaptation of parent–child interaction therapy for Puerto Rican families: A preliminary study. *Family Process, 45,* 205–222.

McCabe, K., & Yeh, M. (2009). Parent–child interaction therapy for Mexican Americans: A randomized clinical trial. *Journal of Clinical Child and Adolescent Psychology, 38*(5), 753–759.

McCabe, K. M., Yeh, M., Garland, A. F., Lau, A. S., & Chavez, G. (2005). The GANA program: A tailoring approach to adapting parent–child interaction therapy for Mexican Americans. *Education and Treatment of Children, 28,* 111–129.

McCabe, K., Yeh, M., Lau, A., & Argote, C. (2012). Parent–child interaction therapy for Mexican Americans: Results of a pilot randomized clinical trial at follow-up. *Behavior Therapy, 43,* 606–618.

McNeil, C. B., Eyberg, S., Hembree-Eisenstadt, T., Newcomb, K., & Funderburk, B.

(1991). Parent–child interaction therapy with behavior problem children: General-ization of treatment effects to the school setting. *Journal of Clinical Child Psychology, 20,* 140–151.

McNeil, C. B., & Hembree-Kigin, T. L. (2010). *Parent–child interaction therapy* (2nd ed.). New York: Springer.

Milner, J. S. (1994). Assessing physical child abuse risk: The child abuse potential inven-tory. *Clinical Psychology Review, 14,* 547–583.

Niec, L. N., Hemme, J. M., Yopp, J. M., & Brestan, E. V. (2005). Parent–child interaction therapy: The rewards and challenges of a group format. *Cognitive and Behavioral Practice, 12,* 113–125.

Nixon, R. D. V. (2001). Changes in hyperactivity and temperament in behaviourally disturbed preschoolers after parent–child interaction therapy (PCIT). *Behaviour Change, 18,* 168–176.

O'Connor, E. E., Collins, B. A., & Supplee, L. (2012). Behavior problems in late child-hood: The roles of early maternal attachment and teacher-child relationship trajec-tories. *Attachment and Human Development, 14*(3), 265–288.

Ondersma, S. J., Chaffin, M. J., Mullins, S. M., & LeBreton, J. M. (2005). A brief form of the Child Abuse Potential Inventory: Development and validation. *Journal of Clinical Child and Adolescent Psychology, 34,* 301–311.

Patterson, G. R. (1982). *Coercive family process.* Eugene, OR: Castalia.

Pincus, D. B., Santucci, L. C., Ehrenreich, J., & Eyberg, S. M. (2008). The implementa-tion of modified parent–child interaction therapy for youth with separation anxiety disorder. *Cognitive and Behavioral Practice, 15,* 118–125.

Radloff, L. S. (1977). The CES-D Scale: A self-report depression scale for research in the general population. *Applied Psychological Measurement, 1,* 385–401.

Reynolds, C. R., & Kamphaus, R. W. (2004). *BASC: Behavior Assessment System for Chil-dren: Manual.* Circle Pines, MN: American Guidance Service.

Schuhmann, E. M., Foote, R., Eyberg, S. M., Boggs, S., & Algina, J. (1998). Parent–child interaction therapy: Interim report of a randomized trial with short-term mainte-nance. *Journal of Clinical Child Psychology, 27,* 34–45.

Thomas, R., & Zimmer-Gembeck, M. J. (2011). Accumulating evidence for parent–child interaction therapy in the prevention of child maltreatment. *Child Development, 82*(1), 177–192.

Thomas, R., & Zimmer-Gembeck, M. J. (2012). Parent–child interaction therapy: An evi-dence-based treatment for child maltreatment. *Child Maltreatment, 17*(3), 253–266.

Timmer, S. G., Borrego, J., Jr., & Urquiza, A. J. (2002). Antecedents of coercive interac-tions in physically abusive mother–child dyads. *Journal of Interpersonal Violence, 17*(8), 836–853.

Timmer, S. G., Ho, L. K. L., Urquiza, A. J., Zebell, N. M., Fernandez y Garcia, E., & Boys, D. (2011). The effectiveness of parent–child interaction therapy with depres-sive mothers: The changing relationship as the agent of individual change. *Child Psychiatry and Human Development, 42,* 406–423.

Timmer, S. G., Urquiza, A. J., Herschell, A. D., McGrath, J. M., Zebell, N. M., Porter, A. L., et al. (2006). Parent–child interaction therapy: Application of an empirically sup-ported treatment to maltreated children in foster care. *Child Welfare, 85*(6), 919–939.

Timmer, S. G., Urquiza, A. J., & Zebell, N. (2006). Challenging foster caregiver–mal-treated child relationships: The effectiveness of parent–child interaction therapy. *Children and Youth Services Review, 28*(1), 1–19.

Timmer, S. G., Urquiza, A. J., Zebell, N. M., & McGrath, J. M. (2005). Parent–child interaction therapy: Application to maltreating parent–child dyads. *Child Abuse and Neglect, 29,* 825–842.

Timmer, S. G., Ware, L. M., Urquiza, A. J., & Zebell, N. M. (2010). The effectiveness of parent–child interaction therapy for victims of interparental violence. *Violence and Victims, 25*(4), 486–503.

Urquiza, A. J., & Blacker, D. M. (2012). Parent–child interaction therapy for sexually abused children. In P. Goodyear-Brown (Ed.), *Handbook of child sexual abuse: Identification, assessment, and treatment.* Hoboken, NJ: Wiley.

Urquiza, A. J., & McNeil, C. B. (1996). Parent–child interaction therapy: An intensive dyadic intervention for physically abusive families. *Child Maltreatment, 1*(2), 134–144.

Werba, B. E., Eyberg, S. M., Boggs, S. R., & Algina, J. (2006). Predicting outcome in parent–child interaction therapy: Success and attrition. *Behavior Modification, 30,* 618–646.

Zayas, L. H., Borrego, J., Jr., & Domenech-Rodríguez, M. (2009). Parenting interventions and Latino families: Research findings, cultural adaptations, and future directions. In F. Villarruel, G. Carlo, J. M. Grau, M. Azmitia, N. Cabrera, and J. Chahin (Eds.), *Handbook of U.S. Latino psychology: Developmental and community based perspectives.* Thousand Oaks, CA: Sage.

10

PCIT with a School-Age Boy Who Experienced Physical Abuse and Neglect

The Case of Christopher J.

Leslie Whitten Baughman

with commentary by Anthony J. Urquiza

BACKGROUND INFORMATION

Christopher J. is a Caucasian boy who was 5 years old when he began treatment at a children's hospital in Northern California. Christopher was referred to treatment by his foster-adoptive father, David, because of aggressive play, deliberate destruction of property, tantrums, oppositional and defiant behaviors, bedtime refusal, and frequent nightmares. Christopher had not received previous mental health services.

At age 4, Christopher was removed from his biological parents by child protective services owing to physical abuse, general neglect, substance abuse in the home, and severe domestic violence. Christopher was initially placed in foster care with a potential adoptive family; however, after 8 months, his behaviors resulted in the loss of that placement. Christopher was then placed in the foster-adoptive home of Steven and David, a Caucasian homosexual couple who had no other children.

ASSESSMENT AND TREATMENT PLANNING

Clinical Interview

At the onset of treatment, a clinical interview was conducted with Christopher's caregivers. Steven and David reported that Christopher had been in their home for almost 4 months and that his behaviors seemed to be worsening. Steven focused heavily on Christopher's negative behaviors, while David pointed out positive moments and argued that Steven had unrealistic expectations for a 5-year-old child. Christopher played roughly with his toys and was often intentionally destructive, such as deliberately crashing his tricycle into furniture. He frequently refused to listen, acting as if he did not hear commands, and his behaviors would intensify if his caregivers attempted discipline. He frequently used physical aggression with his peers, such as grabbing, pushing, and hitting. At bedtime, Christopher would extend the nighttime routine by dawdling and refusing to comply with basic tasks. Once put to bed, he would get up repeatedly over the next several hours. He also experienced nightmares several times a week. It was noted that Christopher could be very loving and kind, but if he did not get his way he would engage in severe temper tantrums that included hitting, throwing objects, kicking walls, and screaming. While Steven wanted to let Christopher "cry it out," David would frequently feel guilty and give in to Christopher's demands. This conflict and others about parenting were causing stress in Steven and David's relationship. Steven shared his fears that Christopher's behaviors would continue to worsen and confided that he was unsure about continuing with the adoption. David felt confident that Christopher's behaviors could be improved and wanted them to move forward with adopting Christopher.

Dyadic Parent–Child Interactive Coding System Observation

The Dyadic Parent–Child Interaction Coding System (DPICS) observational assessment session was conducted with Christopher and each caregiver individually. During the first, child-directed segment of each caregiver's DPICS session, both were independently observed to be highly directive toward Christopher despite instructions to follow the child's lead. When the play activity was changed in the second portion of the observation and the caregiver was instructed to lead, Christopher verbally protested with each parent and continued with his own play. A difference in parenting styles was observed at this point. During Steven's session, he became irritated with Christopher's defiance and raised his voice while repeating commands. During David's session, when faced with the same defiance, he quickly relented and engaged in Christopher's choice of play. With both Steven and David, when the cleanup instructions were given, Christopher verbally protested and refused to put the toys away. Steven responded by becoming angry and giving numerous threats of consequences, although he did not follow through on any of these threats. During David's session, he attempted to model how to clean up for Christopher, but eventually put away all of the toys by himself.

Objective Measures

As part of the assessment, the following objective assessment measures were administered: the Eyberg Child Behavior Inventory (ECBI; Eyberg & Pincus, 1999) and the Child Behavior Checklist (CBCL, 1½–5 years; Achenbach & Rescorla, 2000), both of which assess the severity of children's behavioral problems; the short form of the Parenting Stress Index (PSI; Abidin, 1995), which assesses three sources of stress for the parent: parental distress, dysfunction in the parent–child relationship, and difficult child behavior; and the Trauma Symptom Checklist for Young Children (TSCYC; Briere et al., 2001), a measure of the severity of children's trauma-related symptoms.

Each caregiver completed his own set of measures; however, the outcomes were virtually identical. The following problem areas were identified on the ECBI: table manners, obeying directions, oppositionality, verbal expression, property destruction, and interrupting others. The CBCL yielded scores that were approaching significance in the following areas: withdrawal, somatic complaints, developmental problems, and oppositional defiant problems. The Difficult Child scale on the PSI was elevated, and TSCYC scores were within normal limits. Although some scales were elevated, both caregivers provided relatively few clinically significant elevations on the measures compared to their verbal reports and the DPICS observations conducted during the assessment. It is important to note that the Defensive Responding scale on the PSI was significant for both caregivers, indicating that their written responses on this measure may not have been accurately reported.

Based on the information gathered during the clinical assessment, Christopher was given the diagnosis of disruptive behavior disorder not otherwise specified. Parent–child interaction therapy (PCIT) was recommended to address Christopher's challenging behaviors.

COURSE OF TREATMENT

Child-Directed Interaction Teaching Session

Steven and David met with the clinician for the child-directed interaction (CDI) teaching session. Christopher was not present so as to reduce distraction and allow Steven and David a good opportunity to ask questions and fully understand the information provided. The teaching session addressed key PCIT concepts and how specifically to apply the techniques to Christopher's behaviors. In addition, skills specific to the conduct of PCIT with traumatized children were introduced to help manage Christopher's affective dysregulation (Urquiza, Zebell, Timmer, McGrath, & Whitten, 2011). This discussion included describing and demonstrating the PRIDE skills (Praise, Reflection, Imitation, Description, and Enjoyment), as well as when and how to implement the following techniques: rules (establishing expectations in advance), modeling desired behavior (demonstrating appropriate behaviors), transitional warnings (verbally anticipating a change in routine), when–then/if–then prompts (providing a verbal statement about cause and effect of expected behaviors and consequences), redoing (providing an opportunity to complete an action correctly), choices (offering two options that the caregiver has preselected), and calming exercises (practicing techniques to manage emotions).

David presented as interested and motivated to begin using the therapeutic techniques, while Steven appeared disengaged and did not ask any questions. The clinician's attempts to engage Steven through the use of motivational enhancement techniques (Miller & Rollnick, 2012) were unsuccessful. When the PCIT homework was discussed, David agreed to practice the skills with Christopher for 5 minutes every day as prescribed. Steven stated that his work schedule was inconsistent, but that he would "try" to practice consistently. When the clinician acknowledged Steven's ambivalence, he became noticeably withdrawn and repeated that he would "give it a try."

CDI Coaching Sessions

PCIT is typically provided to one caregiver and one child at a time; however, because of concerns about Christopher losing this placement, it was decided that services would be provided to both Steven and David concurrently. Given Steven's evident resistance to treatment, efforts were made for him to participate in the more structured clinic-based sessions. He cited conflicts with his work schedule and requested in-home services instead. David agreed to attend weekly clinic-based sessions, while Steven agreed to participate in weekly in-home sessions, resulting in Christopher receiving PCIT services twice per week.

In-home sessions were provided by a different clinician from the children's hospital; however, it is possible for a primary treating clinician to provide this service depending on the clinician's availability. In-home PCIT appears to produce comparable results to clinic-based PCIT (Masse & McNeil, 2008) and may enhance the effectiveness of clinic-based PCIT services (Timmer, Zebell, Culver, & Urquiza, 2010). Without a two-way mirror and electronic communication devices, in-home clinicians do their best to coach the parent inconspicuously from the same room as the parent and child. Typically the parent and child engage in play while the clinician sits near or behind the parent and coaches in a quiet tone, so as to reduce any distraction to the play. Although the child may initially comment on the presence of the clinician, as in clinic-based sessions when the child hears a voice in the parent's earpiece, the child quickly forgets about the clinician and readily engages in play.

CDI Coaching Sessions 1–3: Clinic-Based with David

The initial coaching sessions in home, as well as clinic based, focused on building the caregivers' use of the "do" skills using the PRIDE acronym, without focusing too heavily on their use of the "don't" skills (avoid using questions, commands, or criticism). Christopher enjoyed the positive and individual attention he was receiving during both the in-home and clinic-based PCIT sessions.

David was highly responsive to PCIT coaching and quickly began to acquire and generalize the basic skills. Christopher started including David in his play, frequently leaned into David, and voluntarily shared toys with him. When the clinician asked about the 5 minutes of daily at-home PCIT practice with Christopher, David consistently reported that he was able to practice 5 to 7 days each week. Furthermore, he and Christopher were both enjoying the play time together.

During an early coaching session, Christopher began crashing the toy cars into each other. David seemed to want to correct the loud and rough play; however, he was coached to model more appropriate behaviors. The modeling desired behaviors technique, involving slow-motion play, was introduced to allow the fun of the crashes without the recklessness of slamming cars into each other. David was coached to briefly talk about his play, slowing his voice as if he was in a slow-motion movie scene and making the play exciting by demonstrating a slow motion crash: "Oh, that looks like fun! I'm going to crash my cars too. I'm going to do it in sloooow moootionnnn." Then David was instructed to gently and slowly touch his car to another, triggering an exaggerated slow motion reaction that included flying the car into the air and using a controlled motion to flip it carefully end over end and land on the play table. Christopher loved this idea and immediately began crashing his cars in slow motion and imitating David's voice and words. David looked proud when Christopher imitated his actions. Later in the session, Christopher resumed his aggressive play and David was coached to simply say to himself, "Slooooow mmmooooootion," while modeling the technique with his car. Christopher immediately shifted back to slow-motion play without further prompting. David recognized how modeling and playfulness could easily be used to redirect Christopher, rather than engaging in a negative power struggle. David later reported that he was having success, at home and in public, using this type of redirection with Christopher.

Given Christopher's reported and observed difficulties with transitioning between activities, it was decided that the transitional warning technique would be used. Prior to the end of the PCIT session, a warning would be provided: "You have 2 more minutes to play, and then playtime will be over." The first time this technique was used, Christopher verbally protested and began to tantrum. Attention was not given to his tantrum. Two minutes later David was coached to announce that playtime was over and to begin putting the toys away. When the warning was given during the following session, Christopher looked concerned and asked, "Are we coming back again?" David assured him that they would return the following week, and Christopher remained calm. David was coached to praise Christopher for staying calm and to rub his back gently to reinforce his new behavior. At the next session, Christopher responded to the warning by stating in a disappointed voice, "OK," and he joined in when David began to put the toys away. David was coached to praise Christopher enthusiastically for helping to clean up. David saw how preparing Christopher for changes in his routine eased the transitions and reduced negative behaviors. David was encouraged to use transitional warnings with Christopher any time he anticipated a change in Christopher's routine, for example, "Five minutes left to play and then it will be time to get into the bath." The following week, David reported that this technique had significantly reduced the power struggles they were experiencing at home.

During one coaching session, Christopher became upset that the toy train would not stay on the track while pulling it up a bridge. The calming technique was used to teach Christopher how to calm himself when frustrated. David was coached to acknowledge Christopher's feelings, "You look upset," and to demonstrate adaptive coping skills: "When I get upset, it helps me to take a deep breath, like this [modeled taking a deep breath] and count to 5 [slowly]. One, two, three, four, five." Christopher looked at David with a curious expression. David was coached to invite Christopher to try the skills with him, "We can do it together. Deep breath [demonstrated a deep breath]. One, two, three, four, five." Christopher joined in and even counted along with David. The clinician then instructed David to praise Christopher for calming himself. Later in the session, David was coached to create a situation where he could again model coping skills. He pretended to have difficulty constructing a Lego building, as this had been a problem for Christopher at home earlier that day. David paused and stated, "I'm getting mad cause these pieces aren't working the way I want. I'm gonna take a deep breath and count to 5." Christopher smiled and happily joined in with a deep breath and counting. A few minutes later, Christopher was unable to get his own Legos to fit together. His body tightened as if he was about to yell and throw the toys as he had at home earlier that day, but then he paused, took a deep breath and slowly counted to 5. David praised Christopher heartily for using the calming skills. Christopher was proud of himself and sat up straight and smiled at David.

CDI Coaching Sessions 1–3: In-Home with Steven

In-home coaching sessions with Steven were challenging, as he appeared uncomfortable and rarely implemented coaching recommendations. The clinician attempted a variety of coaching styles, from nondirective ("He's really being patient with that difficult toy!") to specific ("Tell Christopher, 'I'm proud of you for staying so calm when that toy isn't working the way you want it to.'"), yet Steven continued to play his own way with Christopher, paying no attention to the coaching directives. Although Christopher enjoyed the PCIT sessions with Steven, he was observed to spend most of the time playing independently, refusing to involve Steven in his activities and at times turning his back to Steven.

The clinician asked specifically about completion of the 5 minutes of daily PCIT homework, which revealed that Steven had not been practicing. Steven provided numerous explanations for why he had not done the work with Christopher: he was too busy, he forgot, and he did not want to reward Christopher's negative behaviors from earlier in the day. The clinician addressed each of these issues in an attempt to problem-solve and break through Steven's resistance, including scheduling a specific time to practice, setting a reminder on Steven's mobile phone, and reminding Steven that playtime serves a valuable therapeutic purpose and that it should never be removed to punish negative behaviors.

At the third coaching session, Steven continued to struggle with acquiring the PRIDE skills. He had yet to complete one 5-minute homework play-time session with Christopher, his use of the PCIT skills had not improved, and Christopher's behaviors with Steven remained unchanged. Steven continued to refuse the clinician's coaching suggestions and appeared irritated by any prompting or feedback. When this resistance was discussed, Steven stated that he was uncomfortable being told what to say and that he disagreed with the concept of following Christopher's lead during the therapy session, stating, "That's what the problem is! He is already in control too much of the time." Attempts to engage Steven by providing a treatment rationale were unsuccessful. Steven was reminded that the first phase of treatment focuses on following the child's lead so as to strengthen the parent–child relationship, and that the parent leads in the second phase of treatment when addressing compliance issues. Following this session, Steven left a voicemail for the clinician stating that his work schedule had changed and that he was no longer able to participate in PCIT sessions. Attempts to speak with Steven about this withdrawal from treatment were unsuccessful.

Following Steven's seeming withdrawal from services, the clinician contacted David to inquire about his own motivation to continue with PCIT. David reported that Steven was never "on board" with treatment and that Steven did not see the value in continuing. David added that he, himself, was very happy with PCIT and that he was able to see a difference in Christopher's behaviors. David indicated that he was highly motivated to continue PCIT services despite Steven's withdrawal. In-home services were offered to David as an adjunct to the clinic-based sessions; however, he declined, as he felt it would be irritating to Steven and add stress to their relationship. Per the family's request, in-home services were discontinued, and weekly clinic-based sessions with David and Christopher continued.

CDI Coaching Sessions 4–7: Clinic-Based with David

As coaching of the PRIDE skills progressed, emphasis was placed on reducing David's attention to Christopher's negative behaviors and decreasing his use of the "don't" skills. During the fourth coaching session, Christopher began making noises as if he was passing gas. He made the noise with his mouth, giggled, and then looked to see David's reaction. When David gave him a disapproving look, Christopher began giggling harder and proceeded to make more inappropriate noises. The clinician pointed out that Christopher was looking for a reaction and, based on the increase in his behaviors, David's reaction was reinforcing the behavior. Because Christopher was neither destructive nor dangerous, it could safely be ignored. However, due to Christopher's history of neglect, he might not have understood that removal of attention was directly linked to his behaviors.

David was coached to use a when–then statement while ignoring Christopher's noises so that Christopher would have a clear understanding of what he could do to reclaim David's attention. The clinician coached David by saying: "Look at your own toys and avoid looking at, talking to, or giving Christopher any reaction in response to the noises. Say to yourself, as if you can't see him, 'When Christopher uses his big-boy voice, I will play with him again.' Now, make your play interesting and describe to yourself what you're doing." David appeared uncomfortable, but was cooperative with the coaching. Christopher responded by increasing his noises and pulling on David's shirt to gain his attention. Although Christopher did not appear to notice, David was clearly upset and wiped tears from his eyes. The clinician acknowledged that David might feel like he is abandoning Christopher, and assured him that this temporary withdrawal would not be detrimental to Christopher or to their relationship. After several more unsuccessful attempts to gain David's attention, Christopher looked disappointed and stated, "OK, I'll stop making fart noises!" David was immediately coached to make eye contact with Christopher and praise him for using his "big-boy voice." Later in the same session, Christopher resumed his inappropriate noises, but this time David only had to look away briefly and Christopher immediately ceased the negative attention-seeking behavior.

At the end of the fourth coaching session, the clinician addressed David's ambivalence about removing his attention from Christopher for negative behaviors. David stated that at first it was very difficult because he did not want Christopher to think that he was abandoning him the way his biological parents had done. David added that once he saw how quickly Christopher's behaviors changed and how he did not seem damaged by the removal of attention, he felt better. He noted feeling very positive about using the ignoring technique after seeing Christopher quickly change his behavior the second time he implemented it.

By the end of the seventh CDI coaching session, David was approaching mastery of the PRIDE skills and, despite reportedly practicing the homework consistently, Christopher's negative behaviors at home and school persisted. The clinician recommended a collateral session with David and Steven so that this concern could be addressed without Christopher present.

Collateral Session

Although Steven was invited to participate in the collateral session, only David attended. David reported that Christopher had been doing very well at home and at school, but that for unknown reasons several times a week his negative behaviors would return. The clinician inquired about factors that may be contributing to Christopher's inconsistent progress, such as inconsistencies at home or trauma reminders. David reported that Steven continued to be unsupportive of treatment and that he frequently contradicted and undermined David in front of Christopher. David also shared concerns about Steven's ability to manage his anger, stating that he would frequently yell at Christopher for minor misbehaviors. Psychoeducation was provided around Christopher's history of trauma and early childhood maltreatment. Specifically, the clinician pointed out that Steven's yelling could be triggering memories of past trauma for Christopher. The impact of neglect, domestic violence, and physical abuse on young children was discussed in detail. David felt strongly about protecting Christopher from reexperiencing any trauma and was motivated to address his concerns with Steven. David additionally confided that after 14 years together, he and Steven were considering separating owing to the stress of Christopher's behaviors and their conflicts over parenting practices. The clinician provided resources and referrals for couples counseling.

Following the collateral session, the clinician contacted David to follow up. David reported that he spoke to Steven about the dynamics that were triggering Christopher's trauma reactions. Steven and David decided that they would no longer share parenting responsibilities and that David would be the primary disciplinarian. This agreement was a further extension of the current parenting roles, as David was already the primary caregiver since Steven was frequently away from home because of his work schedule. Steven agreed either to remove himself from the situation or remain silent, allowing David to manage Christopher's behaviors as he saw fit. Although Steven was not always happy with how David was managing Christopher's behaviors, he acknowledged that Christopher was more cooperative with David. It was later reported that the shift in parenting roles had, surprisingly, reduced the stress in their relationship and that Christopher's behaviors were improving.

CDI Coaching Sessions 8–11: Clinic-Based with David

Coaching continued in an effort to establish more consistent behavior gains with Christopher and for David to reach mastery of the CDI skills. Steven was reportedly able to continue to manage his anger and avoid conflict with Christopher, and gradual behavior progress was reported for Christopher at home and at school. Although David was not able to demonstrate mastery criteria of the CDI skills, the decision was made to move the family to the second phase of treatment, as David's use of the PRIDE skills was consistently close to mastery criteria, he was observed to generalize the skills with Christopher outside of treatment sessions, and his negative interactions with Christopher were eliminated. Changes were also observed in Christopher, such as reduced negative attention-seeking behaviors, improved emotion regulation, and increased responsiveness to David.

Midtreatment Assessment

The DPCIS and the ECBI assessments were conducted at midtreatment with David and Christopher. ECBI scores indicated a reduction in the number of Christopher's problem behaviors in addition to a reduction in the intensity of those behaviors. The DPICS observation revealed a much warmer relationship between David and Christopher. During the child-directed portion, David was able to follow Christopher's lead and demonstrate the PRIDE skills at high levels. During the caregiver-led segment, Christopher initially resisted the shift in play activities, but soon joined in and followed David's lead. During the cleanup scenario, Christopher had difficulty ending the playtime and was uncooperative with the cleanup; however, his behaviors were more controlled than they were during the pretreatment DPICS observation. Verbal reports indicated that Christopher was no longer destructive, was less defiant and oppositional, and his nightmares had ceased. Although David reported that Christopher's behaviors were much improved, they continued to struggle with effective discipline techniques, as he would tantrum in response to consequences.

Parent-Directed Interaction Teaching Sessions

Both Steven and David were invited to the parent-directed interaction (PDI) teaching sessions; however, only David attended. The PDI teaching session was split into two separate sessions owing to time constraints. The first session focused on how to give effective direct commands, and the second session addressed how to implement appropriate consequences. A rationale for these techniques was provided, and role plays were conducted to help David learn these new skills.

The disciplinary techniques were demonstrated for Christopher during the following session through the use of role plays involving a stuffed animal, referred to as Mr. Bear. Christopher enjoyed watching Mr. Bear go to time-out for misbehavior and seemed to understand the cause and effect of misbehavior and consequences.

PDI Coaching Sessions 1–6

PDI coaching sessions attempt to balance the use of CDI skills with the timing and frequency of direct commands. Although coaching of the PDI/PRIDE skills continued, the clinician purposely introduced a new and exciting toy during one of the sessions. When Christopher grabbed the toy out of David's hands, David was coached to give Christopher a command to return the toy. David was able to calmly give the direct command and, when Christopher did not comply, David followed through with the consequence sequence. Christopher still refused to relinquish the toy and David sent him to the time-out chair. Christopher remained seated, but thrashed and screamed loudly.

In traditional PCIT, the parent is coached to say nothing to the child until he or she sits on the time-out chair and remains there for 3 minutes plus 5 seconds of silence. Due to Christopher's trauma history, he had difficulty regulating his emotions and remaining calm enough to understand how he could get out of the time-out. For this reason it was decided that a prompt would be used to help Christopher understand what behaviors he needed to demonstrate in order for him to return to play. David was coached to use a when–then statement to remind Christopher that he needed to sit quietly before he could come back and comply with the original command. To avoid reinforcing Christopher's screaming, David was coached to avoid eye contact with him and to say, "When Christopher can sit quietly on the time-out chair, I will ask him if he's ready to come back and return the toy." David was then coached to be silent and focus his attention on the toys at the table. While Christopher continued to scream for more than 15 minutes, the clinician helped David to continue ignoring his behavior by prompting David to use some of his own relaxation skills, such as deep breathing. Once per minute, David was coached to repeat the when–then statement out loud to himself. Caution was exercised when making the when–then statement to ensure that it was not too frequent and that it was not in response to any of Christopher's comments, so as to avoid reinforcing Christopher's screaming.

Once Christopher was quiet, David was coached to immediately make eye contact with him and state, "You're quiet and sitting in the chair. Are you ready to come back to the table and hand the toy back to me?" Christopher agreed, returned to the table, and returned the toy to David. Per PCIT protocol, David gave Christopher an unlabled praise, "Thank you," to acknowledge Christopher's compliance, but avoided using enthusiasm or physical praise, such as a hug or a high-five, so as not to reinforce Christopher's choice to go to time-out. Following this praise, David gave Christopher a follow-up command to give him the opportunity to comply without going to time-out. Christopher was immediately compliant with the follow-up command, and David gave him a hug and an enthusiastic labeled praise, "Good job listening right away! You don't have to go to time-out when you do what I ask." When Christopher went to the time-out chair for noncompliance during the following session, he calmed himself within 2 minutes. The next time that Christopher was sent to the time-out chair, he was able to calm himself in under a minute. Christopher had successfully learned how to calm himself so that he could comply with the original command. It is important to note that while the duration of Christopher's time-outs was decreasing, his compliance with commands also was improving and he was being sent to time-out less frequently.

PDI sessions continued to incorporate more challenging demands for Christopher, such as introducing toys that were developmentally challenging, taking turns with a construction activity, and creating unexpected transitions. In addition, the concept of logical consequences was used to teach Christopher about the cause and effect of his actions. For example, if Christopher threw one of his toys in anger, the toy would be taken away. House rules, specific to David and Steven's home, were created for situations in which a logical consequence was not applicable. Three basic house rules were implemented: keep hands and feet to self, use kind words and voice, and respect other people's belongings. For instance, if Christopher yelled or called someone names, he was automatically either sent to his room or lost TV time; no prompts or counting were delivered before the delivery of the consequence. By the sixth PDI coaching session, David was able to consistently give an effective command, and Christopher was compliant with more than 90% of all commands.

TREATMENT COMPLETION

Posttreatment DPICS and behavior measures indicated that treatment goals were met. The DPICS session demonstrated a positive relationship between David and Christopher. In addition, David continued to use the PRIDE skills at high levels, and Christopher was compliant with all commands. Scores on the ECBI were significantly reduced for both the Intensity and Problem scales from pretreatment to posttreatment. In addition, considerable improvement was noted on all composite scales of the CBCL. David reported significant reductions in parental stress, as measured by the PSI, and noted being more confident and consistent in his parenting practices. Christopher was no longer destructive with his toys, tantrums and defiant behaviors were reduced to normal limits, and nightmares were eliminated. Overall, Christopher was much better at regulating his emotions and was able to get along better with peers at school.

Although Steven did not participate in PCIT sessions, near the end of treatment he recognized that Christopher's behaviors had improved significantly with David. Steven reportedly began using some of the PCIT techniques at home by emulating David's behaviors. Christopher's relationship with Steven improved, and Steven gradually became more involved with parenting. David reported that the stress in his relationship with Steven was significantly reduced and they were no longer discussing separation. In the end, Steven and David successfully completed their adoption of Christopher.

COMMENTARY

Although there has been a significant rise in evidence-based treatments over the last two decades, nearly all of these interventions have focused on very discrete problems and behaviors, such as posttraumatic stress symptoms, anxiety symptoms, disruptive behaviors, and/or depressive symptoms (Forte, Timmer, & Urquiza, 2014). Although these interventions have demonstrated efficacy and effectiveness for their targeted mental health problems, additional case issues often make it difficult to deliver these interventions in accordance with the prescribed intervention protocol. This is primarily due to the perception that treatment developers require strict adherence to intervention protocols in order for the intervention to work. As a result, many practitioners perceive evidence-based treatments as rigid, inflexible, and not easily adaptable to the unique characteristics of clients. Furthermore, this perceived inflexibility fails to meet the unique and specific needs of their clients, thus resulting in less than expected treatment gains. The product of this apparent dichotomy is that treatment developers have become overly concerned with fidelity in the delivery of their intervention, while clinicians want the freedom to adjust the intervention to their client's needs.

The case of Christopher, David, and Steven provides an excellent example of several issues involved in delivering PCIT, a highly structured evidence-based treatment that often utilizes a session-by-session treatment manual, specific standardized assessment measures, and a presession assessment, and highlights some of the ways in which an intervention can be "tailored" to a client's unique needs. Kendall, Gosch, Furr, and Sood (2008) argue convincingly that making changes to an intervention protocol is a vital process in its practical delivery. While making any type of treatment change increases the risk that aspects of the intervention may become diluted or less effective, Kendall et al. (2008) suggest that developing the proposed change within the intervention's conceptual framework may sustain its effectiveness. Within the case of Christopher, David, and Steven, there were several important changes that highlight this approach.

PCIT with a Child and Substitute Caregivers

Although PCIT was developed with biological parents and their children (Eyberg, 2004), research over the last decade highlights the value of PCIT with several different types of substitute parents/caregivers (Timmer, Urquiza, Herschell, et al., 2006; Timmer, Urquiza, & Zebell, 2006). In the case of Christopher, he was placed in the home of David and Steven as a foster child, with the potential for this to transition to an adoptive placement. Because many children in the child welfare system have disruptive behavior problems, delivering PCIT to enhance the quality of the parent–child relationship, improve parenting skills, and decrease child behavior problems increases the stability of the placement.

Treating Both Parents/Caregivers

The PCIT treatment protocol describes the delivery of the intervention with one parent and one child. However, in this case, the PCIT therapist decided that there could be an increase in the intervention potency by conducting sessions with both parents concurrently. When there is a need to generate rapid treatment gains (i.e., quickly increase child compliance), this is an important clinical decision that can sustain a potentially fragile foster placement. Involving both caregivers in treatment, and having the child be involved in sessions with both caregivers, may prompt a more rapid change in the child's behavioral problems.

Conducting In-Home Treatment Sessions

In addition to increasing the frequency of treatment sessions and having both parents concurrently involved in treatment, it was decided that PCIT sessions with one of the caregivers would take place in the family's home. Delivering in-home PCIT sessions is a new and promising development (Masse & McNeil, 2008; Timmer et al., 2010), with research suggesting that PCIT can be as effective when treatment is delivered in the home as when delivered in a clinic. The clinician in this case attempted to address Steven's struggles in attending clinic-based treatment sessions by shifting to in-home sessions in the hope that he might be more willing to engage in treatment.

The "Modeling Desired Behaviors" Technique

Although not specifically described in PCIT manuals, the process of enhancing Christopher's ability to regulate his play through a "slow-motion" play interaction (i.e., modeling desired behaviors) is a thoughtful technique that is well within the general conceptualization of PCIT (e.g., behavioral and social learning frameworks). Consistently utilized by a parent, this technique can be tremendously valuable in directing a child's behavior.

Transitional Warning Technique

Many children have difficulty with transition, especially children who have experienced consistently unstable, chaotic, and impulsive family environments (such as children in foster care). The clinician in this PCIT case appears familiar with this behavior and has incorporated the "transitional warning technique" into the treatment sessions. This simple technique enhances the predictability of the interaction for Christopher and provides a useful reminder for the caregiver that transitions may be difficult for the child.

Calming Techniques

Among the difficulties often found with children in the child welfare system are problems associated with regulating affect and/or issues with impulsivity/

agitation. Although the focus of PCIT is directed toward behavior management, and teaching emotion regulation skills is not part of the standard protocol, the basic strategy of coaching caregivers to use specific relaxation/calming strategies in session is a highly effective mechanism to teach/train both caregivers and children in the use of these techniques. In this case, the clinician prompted David to teach Christopher several types of relaxation strategies (e.g., deep breathing, counting), and both David and Christopher practiced these skills in session.

When–Then Statements

Various when–then statements (i.e., verbally asserting the consequence of a child's expected behavior) can be a valuable strategy to help gain a child's compliance. The structure of a when–then statement may aid the child in verbally mediated learning of a contingent response, potentially helping the child acquire a better understanding of the consequences of his or her actions.

Summary

This case presentation provides an excellent illustration that learning the basic skills to be a PCIT therapist (i.e., skills described within treatment manuals) is merely the first step toward mastery of the intervention. Continued skill acquisition, education, and experience can help a therapist tailor specific treatment sessions to the client's needs and, therefore, become a more effective PCIT therapist (Urquiza, Zebell, & Blacker, 2009).

REFERENCES

Abidin, R. R. (1995). *Parenting Stress Index—Professional manual* (3rd ed.). Odessa, FL: Psychological Assessment Resources.

Achenbach, T. M., & Rescorla, L. (2000). *Manual for the ASEBA Preschool Forms and Profiles.* Burlington: University of Vermont, Research Center for Children, Youth and Families.

Briere, J., Johnson, K., Bissada, A., Damon, L., Crouch, J., Gil, E., et al. (2001). The Trauma Symptom Checklist for Young Children (TSCYC): Reliability and association with abuse exposure in a multi-site study. *Child Abuse and Neglect, 25,* 1001–1014.

Eyberg, S. M. (2004). The PCIT story—part one: The conceptual foundation of PCIT. *The Parent–Child Interaction Therapy Newsletter, 1,* 1–2.

Eyberg, S. M., & Pincus, D. (1999). *Eyberg Child Behavior Inventory and Sutter–Eyberg Student Behavior Inventory—Revised: Professional manual.* Odessa, FL: Psychological Assessment Resources.

Forte, L. A., Timmer, S. G., & Urquiza, A. J. (2014). Brief history of evidence-based practices. In A. J. Urquiza & S. G. Timmer (Eds.), *Evidence-based approaches for the prevention and treatment of child maltreatment.* New York: Springer.

Kendall, P. C., Gosch, E., Furr, J. M., & Sood, E. (2008). Flexibility within fidelity. *Journal of the Academy and Child and Adolescent Psychiatry, 47,* 987–993.

Masse, J. J., & McNeil, C. B. (2008). In-home parent–child interaction therapy: Clinical considerations. *Child and Family Behavior Therapy, 30,* 127–135.

Miller, W. R., & Rollnick, S. (2012). *Motivational interviewing: Helping people change* (3rd ed.). New York: Guilford Press.

Timmer, S. G., Urquiza, A. J., Herschell, A., McGrath, J., Zebell, N., Porter, A., et al. (2006). Parent–child interaction therapy: Application of an empirically supported treatment to maltreated children in foster care. *Child Welfare, 85,* 919–940.

Timmer, S. G., Urquiza, A. J., & Zebell, N. (2006). Challenging foster caregiver–maltreated child relationships: The effectiveness of parent–child interaction therapy. *Children and Youth Services Review, 28,* 1–19.

Timmer, S. G., Zebell, N. M., Culver, M. A., & Urquiza, A. J. (2010). Efficacy of adjunct in-home coaching to improve outcomes in parent–child interaction therapy. *Research on Social Work Practice, 20,* 36–45.

Urquiza, A. J., Zebell, N. M., & Blacker, D. (2009). Innovation and integration: Parent–child interaction therapy as play therapy. In A. D. Drewes (Ed.), *Blending play therapy with cognitive-behavioral therapy: Evidence-based and other effective treatments and techniques.* New York: Wiley.

Urquiza, A., Zebell, N., Timmer, S., McGrath, J., & Whitten, L. (2011). *PCIT: Sample course of treatment manual for traumatized children.* Unpublished manuscript.

11

PCIT with a Preschool-Age Boy Exposed to Domestic Violence and Maternal Depression

The Case of Jeremy S.

Dawn M. Blacker

with commentary by Anthony J. Urquiza

BACKGROUND INFORMATION

Jeremy S., a 4-year-old Caucasian boy, and his mother, Ms. Smith, were referred for parent–child interaction therapy (PCIT) by Jeremy's pediatrician following extreme disruptive behaviors in the waiting room at a doctor's appointment. Ms. Smith had significant difficulty managing Jeremy's challenging behaviors. Jeremy would hit, kick, and call his mother names when angry and/or when she attempted to set limits. He also displayed difficulty separating from her, refusing to leave her side. There was a family history of chronic and severe domestic violence. During one incident, Jeremy witnessed his father stab his mother with a knife. Jeremy's father was incarcerated at the time of referral because of parole violations, and Ms. Smith had full custody of Jeremy and his older sister, Julia. Jeremy was not attending preschool owing to his disruptive behaviors, and he had not received previous mental health treatment.

ASSESSMENT AND TREATMENT PLANNING

Dyadic Parent–Child Interaction Coding System Observation

Due to standard 50-minute sessions, the intake assessment was conducted over several appointments. Jeremy presented as a quiet and sullen boy. For the first appointment, he refused to separate from his mother to allow for individual interviews. As a result, the pretreatment dyadic parent–child interaction coding system (DPICS) observation was conducted at the first session. During the first 5 minutes, when the parent is instructed to follow the child's lead in play, Ms. Smith spoke little and was passive in her level of engagement. She offered no praise, only two reflections, and seven descriptions. Jeremy was bossy and demanding throughout the first portion of the observation. During the second portion, when the parent is asked to direct session activities, Ms. Smith gave many commands. Jeremy complied with her direction to change the activity; however, he complained and began playing with a different toy than the one she chose. During the "cleanup" scenario, Jeremy complied and put away the toys, but he repeatedly asked to play with a new toy. When his mother told him to remain seated, Jeremy replied, "I hate you!"

Ms. Smith described Jeremy's behavior during the observation as better than what he exhibits at home. She appeared tearful several times during the discussion and stated that she was overwhelmed by Jeremy's behavior. The clinician validated Ms. Smith's concerns, praised her for bringing Jeremy to the session, and informed her that PCIT should help both her and Jeremy. However, the clinician also cautioned that there may be significant challenges during treatment, including Jeremy's behaviors temporarily becoming more intense when the skills are first implemented. Ms. Smith appeared motivated and came to the next assessment session having completed standardized assessment measures provided to her at the end of the first session.

Clinical Interview

The completion of the clinical interview during the second session found that Ms. Smith's pregnancy with Jeremy was typical and he was born full term. Jeremy met all his developmental milestones on time, with the exception of some delays in his verbal expression. He was an energetic, impulsive, and moody toddler; however, the domestic violence in the home was most severe during his toddler years. Jeremy witnessed his father's emotionally and physically abusive behavior daily. When Jeremy was 3 years old, his father was arrested for assault against Ms. Smith and sent to the county jail. The financial impact was significant, and Ms. Smith was struggling to meet their basic needs. She had little social support, was estranged from her parents, and had no siblings. Overall, there were multiple stressors in Ms. Smith's life, including Jeremy's challenging behaviors.

During this second assessment session, Jeremy was able to separate more easily from Ms. Smith so that the clinician could administer a cognitive screening instrument, which revealed no significant problems. During administration of the cognitive screener, Jeremy abruptly disclosed that his father would hit his mother, but that it was "a long time ago."

At the end of the second session, the clinician again provided validation and encouragement to Ms. Smith and helped her identify other sources of support (e.g., friends). The therapist affirmed that PCIT should reduce Jeremy's challenging behaviors and provide her with new parenting skills to manage problematic behaviors in the future. Ms. Smith and the clinician determined that treatment goals would be to decrease Jeremy's physical aggression, increase his compliance with commands, and decrease his negative verbalizations. Ms. Smith agreed to come back by herself for the didactic session focused on child-directed interaction (CDI) skills.

Objective Measures

Following the intake assessment, the standardized assessment measures completed by Ms. Smith were scored to assist with further treatment planning and monitoring. The measures included the Eyberg Child Behavior Inventory (ECBI; Eyberg & Pincus, 1999), the Child Behavior Checklist (CBCL; Achenbach & Rescorla, 2000), the Parenting Stress Index (PSI; Abidin, 1995), the Trauma Symptom Checklist for Young Children (TSCYC; Briere, 2005), the Child Abuse Potential Inventory (CAPI; Milner, 1986), and the Brief Symptom Index (BSI; Derogatis, 1993). Overall, results from the CBCL indicated that Jeremy was exhibiting clinically significant externalizing and internalizing problems. He also displayed symptoms of posttraumatic intrusive thoughts, anxiety, and depression according to the TSCYC. The PSI results revealed that Ms. Smith experienced significant stress in her role as a parent and perceived Jeremy as a difficult child. In addition, she described behaviors and attitudes characteristic of individuals at risk for committing child physical abuse on the CAPI and reported on the BSI that she experienced symptoms of somatic complaints, obsessive–compulsive problems, depression, anxiety, and hostility.

Based on the pretreatment DPICS observations, test results, clinical observations, and clinical interviews, Jeremy was diagnosed with disruptive behavior disorder not otherwise specified and anxiety disorder not otherwise specified.

COURSE OF TREATMENT

Child-Directed Interaction Teaching Session

For the CDI didactic, both Jeremy and Ms. Smith attended, as Ms. Smith was unable to obtain childcare for Jeremy. During the session, Jeremy became agitated and began pulling Ms. Smith's hair and hitting her. When she attempted to set limits, he angrily knocked over a chair. The clinician attempted to provide encouragement and suggested that his behavior should improve following implementation of the PRIDE skills (Praise, Reflection, Imitation, Description, and Enjoyment), which were explained in detail. The clinician attempted to normalize Jeremy's behavior within the context of exposure to domestic violence and discussed how his father modeled violent behavior for him. In addition, the possibility that Jeremy's angry outbursts reflect posttraumatic stress reactions was discussed. Jeremy's misbehavior continued throughout the session, making it difficult for Ms. Smith to focus on the material being presented. At the end of the session, Jeremy refused to leave and was carried out by Ms. Smith, who appeared embarrassed and overwhelmed with Jeremy's behavior.

CDI Coaching Sessions

CDI Coaching Sessions 1–5

For the first CDI coaching session, Jeremy was argumentative during play. He often told Ms. Smith, "You're not doing that right!" The clinician coached Ms. Smith to use selective attention and ignore Jeremy's argumentative behavior. Initially, Jeremy appeared confused by Ms. Smith's response, but his argumentative comments soon stopped and he resumed playing. Given the complete lack of praise provided by Ms. Smith during the initial DPICS observation, the clinician made a concerted effort to encourage Ms. Smith to offer more praise during session. The clinician coached her to praise Jeremy for staying in his seat, using his "inside voice," and playing nicely with the toys. This appeared difficult for Ms. Smith, but she implemented the coaching from the clinician nonetheless.

For the second session, Jeremy displayed more appropriate behavior and engaged in a positive manner when Ms. Smith used the PRIDE skills. However, Ms. Smith disclosed to the clinician that she was feeling depressed due to ongoing financial stressors and that she was having difficulty providing positive attention to Jeremy and his sister. She also displayed physical symptoms of depression (e.g., insomnia, increased appetite). The therapist recommended that Ms. Smith seek services for herself and provided several referrals for treatment. The clinician continued to coach Ms. Smith in the selective attention and PRIDE skills, but it was apparent that Ms. Smith was struggling, as she was lethargic and unenthusiastic.

During the opening observation of the third session, it was notable that Ms. Smith was less engaged with Jeremy and used few PRIDE skills. Correspondingly, Jeremy exhibited increased negative attention-seeking behavior. For instance, Jeremy began the play session by using profane language to refer to various toys. The clinician coached Ms. Smith to avoid looking at or saying anything to him and, instead, to play with the toys by herself. Jeremy quickly stopped using profanity, and Ms. Smith was coached to praise Jeremy for his appropriate behavior and language as she reengaged in play with him. At the end of the session, the clinician followed up with Ms. Smith about the referral for her own mental health services. She was unable to connect with a provider during the past week because of time constraints, but agreed to do so before the next session.

As it was noted that Ms. Smith consistently failed to practice the skills at home through the completion of homework, the clinician decided to address this issue during the fourth CDI coaching session. The clinician emphasized the importance of completing the homework to improve her comfort with the skills and ability to implement them effectively. Ms. Smith identified two separate barriers to completing the homework. First, her depression was significantly impairing her functioning. The clinician recommended that Ms. Smith request a psychiatric evaluation to determine whether medication might help decrease her symptoms of depression, and provided referral information. The clinician learned through this discussion that Ms. Smith had not yet sought mental health services for herself as discussed in previous sessions. The clinician attempted to motivate Ms. Smith to seek these services, as she previously agreed, by pointing out her own perception that her mental health concerns were interfering with her ability to control Jeremy's behavior. Second, Ms. Smith discussed how she was withholding the daily homework playtime from Jeremy to punish his problematic behaviors. The clinician informed Ms. Smith that the daily play session was not a reward or a privilege to be used as a consequence. Rather, it was an opportunity for her to improve her relationship with Jeremy and practice the PCIT skills at home, which would improve her ability to control his behaviors. Ms. Smith agreed to no longer use the removal of the daily play session as a discipline tool and implement the daily play session at home regardless of how Jeremy's behaved.

At the beginning of the fifth session, Jeremy insisted on stopping at a drinking fountain on the way to the treatment room. When Ms. Smith refused, Jeremy became enraged and began to hit her and to throw the toys and chairs that were in the hallway. The clinician coached Ms. Smith to use selective attention and limit setting to ensure her safety and that of the clinician. Ms. Smith appeared afraid of Jeremy at various points in the altercation, and the clinician provided encouragement and praise for Ms. Smith's continued use of selective attention. Despite the attempts of Ms. Smith and the clinician to calm Jeremy, he continued to exhibit dangerous and destructive behavior. As a result, the session ended early. During the tantrum, Ms. Smith reported that she had made an appointment to see a psychiatrist for a medication evaluation and felt positive about taking steps to improve her own mental health. The clinician praised Ms. Smith for contacting the psychiatrist and for following through with not allowing Jeremy to have water before the session.

CDI Coaching Sessions 6–11

Ms. Smith began the sixth session by reporting that she saw a psychiatrist and started a trial of an antidepressant. After several weeks, Ms. Smith's mood improved significantly; however, she had not obtained psychological treatment for herself. In addition, her completion of PCIT homework remained inconsistent. Further complicating the situation was the fact that Jeremy's father had been released from jail, and Jeremy was visiting him occasionally.

In addition to the regular coaching of CDI skills, the clinician and Ms. Smith spent time each session problem-solving the barriers that were interfering with her ability to complete homework. Ms. Smith identified various barriers, but the most pressing challenge appeared to change each week. Commonly cited challenges included: difficulty scheduling time for special playtime with Jeremy's sister at home, difficulty deciding which toys to use, and assertions that Jeremy did not wish to participate in special playtime. Plans to overcome the barriers were developed each week, such as scheduling the homework when his sister is in school and designating specific toys as "special playtime toys" that would only be available to Jeremy during special playtime.

Despite Ms. Smith's inconsistency in completing the homework, Jeremy's behavior in sessions improved. Ms. Smith continued to respond well to the ongoing coaching, and Jeremy's mood appeared more positive. Jeremy's physical and verbal aggression toward Ms. Smith was greatly reduced. Jeremy seemed particularly responsive to Ms. Smith's use of reflections and descriptions of his behavior, although he occasionally reacted in a sarcastic way when Ms. Smith provided direct, labeled praise. The clinician coached Ms. Smith simply to ignore his sarcastic comments and continue playing. Selective attention became one of the most effective tools for Ms. Smith, as Jeremy did not like the moments when he lost his mother's attention. When the selective attention technique was employed, Jeremy typically ceased his problematic behavior within seconds. However, even with these noticeable changes in session, Ms. Smith continued to report that Jeremy's behavior at home remained challenging and that he continued to hit her almost daily.

Because of Ms. Smith's inconsistent completion of homework and seeming inability to effectively implement the skills at home, the clinician decided to conduct a collateral session alone with Ms. Smith to address these concerns. During this session, the clinician reiterated the purpose of the homework (e.g., generalization of skills to the home and community, develop a more positive relationship with Jeremy) and the importance of practicing the skills outside of session. To address the physical aggression, the clinician recommended implementing a "no hitting" rule where Jeremy would immediately be placed into an "automatic time-out" if he hit or kicked anyone. Ms. Smith appeared somewhat nervous at the suggestion. She was willing to try using the house rule, but admitted she was concerned that Jeremy's aggressive behavior would escalate with the implementation of this rule. The clinician agreed that his physical aggression might increase, but emphasized that the increase would be temporary and ultimately the aggression should decrease. The clinician and Ms. Smith agreed to explain the rule to Jeremy in session prior to implementation. Last, it was suggested that Ms. Smith begin attending regular individual sessions with a clinician to help her better understand Jeremy's behaviors and address her ongoing hesitation and difficulty implementing the PCIT skills outside of sessions. Due to time constraints, the PCIT clinician was not able to provide Ms. Smith these sessions; however, another clinician at the clinic was assigned specifically to provide her with these one-on-one sessions.

The individual sessions with Ms. Smith initially focused on providing psychoeducation regarding the impact of domestic violence. Although Ms. Smith had previously received this information, the individual sessions allowed a deeper discussion of the material and an examination of how her own experience of domestic violence affected her relationship with Jeremy. She gained a greater respect for how Jeremy's witnessing of the domestic violence influenced the development of his behavioral problems, both through the modeling of violent behavior and posttraumatic stress symptoms. Ms. Smith's hesitation to change the established pattern of interacting with Jeremy (i.e, he was aggressive, she was passive) was a primary topic of discussion. She was able to describe how Jeremy's anger and aggression frightened her, most likely because it reminded her of the domestic violence she experienced. The clinician empathized with Ms. Smith and cautioned that it would take time for Jeremy to learn new ways of interacting with her. However, she was encouraged to be consistent in her delivery of consequences for Jeremy's behaviors, as this consistency offered the most effective route toward reducing his anger and aggression.

The clinician also taught Ms. Smith basic relaxation skills (e.g., controlled breathing) to help manage her own posttraumatic stress symptoms. Since the funding source only allowed treatment for the child, the goal of the individual sessions with Ms. Smith remained focused on assisting Jeremy and could not provide direct treatment for Ms. Smith's own mental health concerns. However, the clinician concurred with the PCIT clinician and encouraged Ms. Smith to initiate her own mental health treatment with a focus on depressive and posttraumatic stress symptoms. Ms. Smith attended a total of seven individual sessions with this clinician, but never initiated her own mental health treatment services throughout the duration of PCIT treatment.

CDI Coaching Sessions 12–15

After conducting the collateral session, and commencing the individual sessions, there was marked improvement in Ms. Smith's completion of homework. For example, between Sessions 12 and 14, she completed the homework six out of seven days, and seven out of seven days, respectively. As a result, Ms. Smith's efficiency in the use of the PRIDE skills improved significantly, and she met the mastery criteria for the PRIDE skills during the 15th session. Jeremy's behavior in session was more calm and gentle.

Although Jeremy did not exhibit aggressive behavior in the clinic, he was still physically aggressive toward Ms. Smith at home. She was not implementing the "no hitting" rule consistently because she was afraid of her son's aggressive reaction, expressing concern that he was "becoming his father." Owing to her increased understanding of trauma-related topics acquired during her individual sessions, Ms. Smith was able to describe herself as experiencing a traumatic stress reaction whenever Jeremy became physically aggressive. The clinician empathized with how difficult it was to implement discipline in response to this behavior while she was experiencing such a reaction; however, the clinician asserted that Ms. Smith's ability to set limits and deliver appropriate consequences was necessary if the aggressive behavior were to be reduced. The clinician explained that the "automatic time-out" rule was designed specifically to address such aggressive behavior. Ms. Smith was receptive to the conversation and agreed to begin implementing the "automatic time-out" in response to her son's aggressive behavior. Subsequent sessions found that Ms. Smith had, indeed, begun using the rule consistently, and Jeremy's physical aggression toward Ms. Smith in the home decreased.

For the midtreatment DPICS observation, Ms. Smith demonstrated a solid understanding of the PRIDE skills, with significant increases in the use of all skills; however, Ms. Smith continued to use indirect commands and she did not consistently praise Jeremy for his compliance with those commands.

Jeremy appeared more engaged with Ms. Smith and demonstrated an increased frequency of compliance when she gave directions. Scores on the ECBI, which was the only measure administered at the midtreatment assessment, demonstrated significant reductions in the intensity of Jeremy's behavioral problems.

Parent-Directed Interaction Teaching Sessions

The parent-directed interaction (PDI) didactic was separated into two treatment sessions as a result of the time limitations. The first session was spent reviewing the concepts of PDI with Ms. Smith and demonstrating the "time-out" procedure. The clinician discussed how the techniques would be used with Jeremy, using some of his more common behavioral problems as examples. The subsequent session was spent teaching Jeremy the time-out procedure with the assistance of a stuffed animal. Specifically, Ms. Smith modeled giving direct and effective commands to the stuffed animal in front of Jeremy and used the time-out sequence for noncompliance. Jeremy was primarily interested in his own play, but would often stop and look at his mother and the stuffed animal as the time-out sequence progressed. This was repeated several times to acquaint Jeremy with the new technique and the consequences involved for noncompliance.

PDI Coaching Sessions

PDI Coaching Sessions 1–8

For the first PDI coaching session, Jeremy was notably compliant with all of Ms. Smith's commands. Ms. Smith provided a number of effective commands, with the assistance of coaching from the clinician, but never reached the point in the sequence when a time-out was delivered. A primary focus of this first session was coaching Ms. Smith to increase her use of labeled praise when Jeremy complied. Her progress throughout the course of the first PDI coaching session was noticeable.

Jeremy was generally compliant for most of the second PDI coaching session, until shortly before the end. After being sent to the time-out chair for refusing to pass Ms. Smith a toy, Jeremy refused to sit in the chair and started yelling profanities. As a result, the clinician coached Ms. Smith to use the "swoop and go" technique, gathering all of the toys and promptly leaving the room. This technique effectively removes all attention and opportunity for play. Jeremy's behavior escalated and he started throwing chairs at the observation window. The clinician consulted with Ms. Smith, and it was determined that Jeremy would lose the privilege of watching his favorite television show for the remainder of the day if he did not sit in the time-out chair. Ms. Smith re-entered the room and delivered the choices to Jeremy, who continued his tantrum and refused to sit in the chair. To remove Jeremy from the situation, the decision was made to end the session and leave the clinic. Jeremy refused to leave, and he was carried out of the clinic by his mother, with assistance from the clinician. Along the way, Jeremy kicked both Ms. Smith and the clinician.

The clinician made a follow-up telephone call later that day to Ms. Smith, who reported that Jeremy's behavior improved when he was in the car. She had followed through with the consequence of not allowing Jeremy to watch his favorite television show, despite Jeremy calling her "mean." Ms. Smith was embarrassed by Jeremy's behavior at the clinic and felt guilty for having such difficulty managing his behavior. She reiterated that Jeremy's aggressive behavior reminded her of his father and resulted in a sudden feeling of fear. The clinician validated Ms. Smith's feelings and praised her for continuing to deliver the necessary consequences even though she felt anxious.

The next five PDI sessions were relatively unremarkable. Although Jeremy was generally compliant in the clinic, Ms. Smith continued to have difficulty using direct commands, and the clinician was required to prompt her to begin the time-out procedure if Jeremy did not comply immediately. When consequences were delivered during these sessions, Jeremy did not show the types of severe responses previously observed.

Following the third PDI session, Ms. Smith was instructed to begin using direct commands and the time-out procedure at home. During the fourth PDI coaching session, house rules, including "keeping hands to self" and "use respectful words," were reviewed with Jeremy and Ms. Smith. The first of these rules targeted elimination of physical aggression and the second was designed to reduce profanity. Violation of these rules resulted in an automatic time-out. By the seventh PDI session, Ms. Smith reported that Jeremy was being placed in fewer time-outs at home and exhibiting less physical aggression. By the eighth PDI session, Ms. Smith was close to mastery in using direct commands, but still needed prompting in using the time-out warning when Jeremy did not immediately comply.

PDI Coaching Sessions 9–15

At the beginning of the ninth PDI session, almost immediately after the clinician arrived in the waiting room to greet Ms. Smith and Jeremy, Jeremy hit his mother in response to a command and was placed into an automatic time-out. Ms. Smith needed little prompting to implement the automatic time-out; however, Jeremy refused to stay in the time-out chair. Ms. Smith quickly implemented a "swoop and go" technique, removing the toys in front of Jeremy in the waiting room. It took approximately 30 minutes for Jeremy to sit in the time-out chair. The clinician provided significant coaching and encouragement to Ms. Smith throughout this period, including praising her for following through and being consistent despite having others in the waiting room witness the sequence. At the conclusion of Jeremy's time-out, Ms. Smith immediately gave him a follow-up direct command and Jeremy ignored her. He was returned to the time-out chair. He remained in the chair for 3 minutes and then complied with the original command, as well as a follow-up command.

The clinician praised Ms. Smith's use of the PCIT skills and noted that she appeared calmer during the episode in the waiting room than during previous behavioral episodes that occurred at the clinic. Ms. Smith admitted to still feeling overwhelmed by Jeremy's disruptive behavior, especially when implementing the time-out procedure. Due to time constraints, the therapist agreed to continue the discussion with Ms. Smith at the next session. The clinician agreed to meet individually with Ms. Smith to discuss her continuing discomfort when delivering consequences for Jeremy's behavioral problems.

At the next session, the clinician reinforced the information regarding the dynamics of domestic violence that Ms. Smith had learned during her individual sessions with the other clinician. Specifically, the discussion centered on identifying how those dynamics and her own posttraumatic stress reactions created barriers that were affecting her ability to deliver discipline consistently. The clinician role-played various scenarios with Ms. Smith for the purpose of presenting her with situations she might encounter. The purpose of these role plays was to allow Ms. Smith to practice her responses to aggressive behavior so as to decrease the likelihood that her trauma-induced reactions would make her unable to determine or implement appropriate consequences. Ms. Smith was thankful to be able to practice these responses and believed they would be helpful the next time Jeremy displayed aggressive behavior.

During the next two PDI sessions, Jeremy was compliant with 100% of Ms. Smith's commands, and she was able to state direct and effective commands 75% of the time with no prompting. In addition, Ms. Smith reported that Jeremy was becoming more compliant at home and only needed time-out warnings 20% of the time before complying with a direct command. Ms. Smith believed she was more assertive at home and was implementing consequences with significantly greater frequency. As a result, Jeremy's physical aggression and use of profanity diminished considerably. The clinician and Ms. Smith jointly decided that sessions would now be conducted every other week to begin the process of working toward treatment discharge.

Jeremy complied with all of Ms. Smith's commands in the clinic during the final two PDI sessions. Ms. Smith continued to complete homework and reported that Jeremy was sent to time-out only once in a span of 4 weeks. She reported no incidents of physical aggression, profanity, or name-calling.

In addition, Ms. Smith demonstrated a solid understanding of both CDI and PDI skills and required minimal coaching from the therapist. During the 14th session, it was mutually decided that the following session would constitute a graduation session from PCIT.

TREATMENT COMPLETION

At the graduation session, Ms. Smith again reported frequent compliance from Jeremy and no new incidents of physical aggression or profanity. For the posttreatment DPICS observation, she provided 13 labeled praises, six behavioral descriptions, and 16 reflections during the initial 5-minute, child-directed portion. When changing activities, Jeremy was responsive to Ms. Smith's direct commands and remained in a positive mood. He also complied with her direct commands to clean up the toys at the end of the observation, and Ms. Smith immediately praised him for complying. The therapist praised Ms. Smith and Jeremy for their progress and completion of treatment.

The clinician asked Ms. Smith to complete the same series of questionnaires given to her during the intake assessment to ascertain any remaining emotional or behavioral concerns and subsequent treatment needs for Jeremy. The results of the questionnaires revealed no significant internalizing or externalizing problems, and Jeremy's posttraumatic stress symptoms were no longer clinically elevated; however, Ms. Smith did report that Jeremy displayed poor social skills, and it was decided that he would attend a social skills group through his school. Despite these concerns about Jeremy's social skills, he was doing well academically and behaviorally in school.

Ms. Smith reported significant improvements in her own mental health on the BSI and a significantly reduced risk for committing child physical abuse, as measured by the CAPI. Although she reported substantially reduced parental stress, some subscales of the PSI remained in the elevated range (i.e., Parental Distress, Dysfunctional Parent–Child Relationship). It appeared that Ms. Smith also believed that there was significant improvement in Jeremy's behavior overall; however, she still perceived their relationship as being stressful. It should be noted that Ms. Smith continued to experience ongoing life stressors (e.g., financial concerns, a conflicted relationship with Jeremy's father, her own mental health concerns). The clinician encouraged her to continue using the PCIT after graduation to continue to improve the parent–child relationship and help reduce her stress. Neither Ms. Smith nor the clinician believed that the remaining stress warranted continued treatment.

Treatment progress was slow due to various barriers, including Ms. Smith's own mental health concerns, inconsistent completion of homework, and lack of consistency in the use of discipline skills largely as a result of Ms.

Smith's previous experience of domestic violence. Because of the complexity of the case, the therapist was required to respond to various issues to ensure that both Jeremy and Ms. Smith would benefit from PCIT. Attempts to address Ms. Smith's mental health symptoms were frequent, and included a referral for a psychiatric medication evaluation, a referral to an outside mental health clinician for her own personal therapy, multiple one-on-one individual sessions with a second agency clinician, and multiple collateral sessions with the PCIT clinician to resolve barriers to treatment. Ongoing psychoeducation about domestic violence and posttraumatic stress symptoms was required, and role plays were used to problem-solve challenging situations in which Ms. Smith's posttraumatic stress reactions interfered with providing discipline. These interventions supplemented the standard process of delivering PCIT treatment and served to increase Jeremy's compliance and decrease his aggressive behavior.

COMMENTARY

PCIT was developed as an intervention for children with various types of disruptive behavior problems, such as defiance, noncompliance, and temper tantrums (Eyberg, 2004). However, it is not uncommon for children presenting for outpatient mental health services to display a combination of mental health concerns that includes disruptive behavior problems and trauma-related symptoms (Valentino, Berkowitz, & Stover, 2010). One of the difficulties of treating a client such as Jeremy, who displayed disruptive behavior problems and trauma-related symptoms, is determining the intervention that is most appropriate to meet his needs: an intervention targeting the defiance and aggression or an intervention to reduce posttraumatic stress and other trauma-related concerns.

Jeremy's case demonstrates an opportunity to possibly address trauma-related symptoms *and* disruptive behavior concurrently. Recently, research has shown that traumatized children may exhibit a significant reduction in trauma-related symptoms as a result of their involvement in PCIT (Mannarino, Lieberman, Urquiza, & Cohen, 2010). This finding, that an intensive behavioral parenting program may result in a reduction of trauma symptoms, may initially be puzzling to some. However, on closer inspection, there are several reasons why traumatized children would benefit from PCIT.

Management of Disruptive Behavior

Many children exposed to violence come from chaotic and dysfunctional families and are consistently exposed to poor and inconsistent parenting, which leads to defiant, oppositional, and aggressive behavior (behaviors that qualify them as an appropriate match for PCIT). Also, for some children, their posttraumatic stress responses are exhibited through defiant and disruptive behaviors. It therefore should be no surprise that helping parents manage their child's disruptive behavior in a positive, consistent, and firm manner, which is an objective of PCIT, should result in a decrease in trauma-related symptoms.

Improved Caregiver–Child Relationship

In addition to the management of challenging child behavior, PCIT fosters a more positive and supportive parent–child relationship. One of the avenues to recovery from any victimization or trauma exposure involves eliciting support from important caregivers. That is, supportive parenting is associated with positive child outcomes in many domains (Greenberg, 1999), especially when a child is required to deal with some type of adverse experience. Therefore, it is essential to sustain a positive parent–child relationship and parental support in order to optimize the child's ability to deal with any adverse or traumatic experience. The combination of parental stress associated with a child's experience of trauma and problematic child symptoms can erode a parent's ability to be supportive, warm, and understanding. One benefit of PCIT is that it provides a mechanism to strengthen the parent–child relationship through coaching of positive affiliative behaviors (e.g., praising, physical affection). Throughout PCIT, there is an emphasis on helping parents to recognize and verbally deliver positive statements to their children (concurrently, there is an emphasis to ignore minor negative and inappropriate behaviors) in an effort to help parents maintain a warm and supportive relationship with their children. It is important to remember that the early foundation of PCIT derives from Sheila Eyberg's (2004) effort to create an intervention that promoted the healthiest parenting style, authoritative parenting (Baumrind, 1966), which includes the combination of nurturing interaction, clear communication, and firm limitsetting.

Parents as Therapists: Supporting Parent–Child Communication

Although there are many perspectives on what exactly constitutes psychotherapy, there is a rich literature describing parents functioning in a supportive, therapeutic-like role with their children (see Guerney, 2000; Hutton, 2004). The central aspects of this type of filial therapy relationship include (1) a positive relationship between a child and parent, (2) a focus on the development of appropriate and safe expression/communication, and (3) the use of play as a central theme (Urquiza, Zebell, & Blacker, 2009). Within

PCIT, parents receive direct instruction on how to engage their children in positive and collaborative play (especially in the first component of PCIT). As a result, typically a warmer, more supportive, and affectionate relationship develops between the parent and child. Often, this includes positive verbal statements and physical affection exhibited by both the parent and the child. Similarly, the focus on safe and effective communication is a central tenet of PCIT. Parents are directed to communicate issues of safety, concern for the child's well-being, and positive regard for all appropriate and nonaggressive/nonhostile interactions. Because play activities are generally perceived by both parent and child as positive and enjoyable, sharing such activities within a PCIT session contributes to the overall positive experience that both parent and child convey toward each other, while strengthening the communication between the dyad.

Management of the Trauma-Exposed Child's Affect

It is well recognized that trauma-exposed young children may have difficulty managing their feelings, particularly in emotionally difficult situations. In addition to developing a more positive and secure parent–child relationship, PCIT can directly address many of the feelings that a child experiences. Consistent throughout common PCIT protocol is the identification of the child's thoughts, feelings, and behaviors. Should a trauma-exposed child experience some type of unpleasant affect, especially related to feelings of anger, frustration, embarrassment, and/or shame, parents are coached to recognize and describe these feelings to the child. As children have the experience of their feelings paired with the label presented by parents, they begin to understand the meaning of the distressing affect, which is one of the first steps to being able to discuss and manage these feelings. As children continue to understand these feelings, parents can help them learn to employ strategies to manage these feelings (e.g., deep breathing, counting, and progressive relaxation). Although not a core feature of PCIT, the clinician can integrate emotion regulation skills training into treatment and have the parent and child practice these skills in session.

Summary

The usefulness of PCIT with young trauma-exposed children who display disruptive behaviors is not to suggest that PCIT is a panacea. As was the case with Jeremy's mother, much of the weight of this intervention falls on the parent's ability to be engaged and motivated to support the child. For Jeremy's mother, her mental health problems (primarily depression) impaired both her capacities and her son's pathway to health. This is a reminder of the value of parent–child dyadic interventions for young children. Overall, PCIT fills a very important and urgent need for young trauma-exposed children who present with significant behavioral disruption. Future efforts to support and enhance the quality of the parent–child relationship, an essential aspect of PCIT, offer an exciting direction for trauma treatment.

REFERENCES

Abidin, R. R. (1995). *The Parenting Stress Index professional manual*. Odessa, FL: Psychological Assessment Resources.

Achenbach, T. M., & Rescorla, L. A. (2000). *Manual for the ASEBA preschool forms and profiles*. Burlington: University of Vermont, Research Center for Children, Youth, and Families.

Baumrind, D. (1966). Effects of authoritative parental control on child behavior. *Child Development, 37*, 887–907.

Briere, J. (2005). *Trauma Symptom Checklist for Young Children: Professional manual*. Odessa, FL: Psychological Assessment Resources.

Derogatis, L. R. (1993). *Brief Symptom Inventory: Administration, scoring, and procedures manual* (3rd ed.). Minneapolis: National Computer Systems.

Eyberg, S. (2004) The PCIT story—Part one: The conceptual foundation of PCIT. *The Parent–Child Interaction Therapy Newsletter, 1*, 1–2.

Eyberg, S. M., & Pincus, D. (1999). *Eyberg Child Behavior Inventory and Sutter–Eyberg Behavior Inventory—Revised: Professional manual*. Odessa, FL: Psychological Assessment Resources.

Greenberg, M.T. (1999). Attachment and psychopathology in childhood. In J. Cassidy & P. R. Shaver (Eds.), *Handbook of attachment: Theory, research, and clinical applications*. New York: Guilford Press.

Guerney, L. (2000). Filial therapy into the 21st century. *International Journal of Play Therapy, 9*, 1–17.

Hutton, D. (2004). Filial therapy: Shifting the balance. *Clinical Child Psychology and Psychiatry, 9*, 1359–1045.

Mannarino, A., Lieberman, A., Urquiza, A., & Cohen, J. (2010). *Evidence-based treatments for traumatized children*. Panel discussion at the 118th annual convention of the American Psychological Association, San Diego, CA.

Milner, J. (1986). *The Child Abuse Potential Inventory manual*. DeKalb, IL: Psytec.

Urquiza, A. J., Zebell, N. M., & Blacker, D. (2009). Innovation and integration: Parent–child interaction therapy as play therapy. In A. D. Drewes (Ed.), *Blending play therapy with cognitive-behavioral therapy: Evidence-based and other effective treatments and techniques*. New York: Wiley.

Valentino, K., Berkowitz, S., & Stover, C. S. (2010). Parenting behaviors and posttraumatic symptoms in relation to children's symptomatology following a traumatic event. *Journal of Traumatic Stress, 23*, 403–407.

Index